IMMUNOLOGY
for Life Scientists

IMMUNOLOGY
for Life Scientists

A Basic Introduction

A Student-centred Learning Approach

LESLEY-JANE EALES

University of Surrey, Guildford, UK

JOHN WILEY & SONS

Chichester • New York • Weinheim • Brisbane • Singapore • Toronto

Content Copyright © 1997 John Wiley & Sons, Ltd,
Baffins Lane, Chichester,
West Sussex PO19 1UD, UK.

Published 1997 by John Wiley & Sons, Ltd

National   01243 779777
International (+44) 1243 779777
e-mail (for orders and customer service enquiries): cs-books@wiley.co.uk
Visit our Home Page on http://www.wiley.co.uk
            or http://www.wiley.com

Other Wiley Editorial Offices

John Wiley & Sons, Inc., 605 Third Avenue,
New York, NY 10158-0012, USA

WILEY-VCH Verlag GmbH, Pappelallee 3,
D-69469 Weinheim, Germany

Jacaranda Wiley Ltd, 33 Park Road, Milton,
Queensland 4064, Australia

John Wiley & Sons (Asia) Pte Ltd, 2 Clementi Loop #02-01,
Jin Xing Distripark, Singapore 129809

John Wiley & Sons (Canada) Ltd, 22 Worcester Road,
Rexdale, Ontario M9W 1L1, Canada

Library of Congress Cataloging-in-Publication Data

Eales, Lesley-Jane.
    Immunology for life scientists : a basic introduction : a student-
centered learning approach / Lesley-Jane Eales.
        p.   cm.
    Includes bibliographical references and index.
    ISBN 0-471-96225-2 (pbk.)
    1. Immunology. 2. Immunopathology. 3. Immunity.   I. Title
QR181.E24   1997
616.07′9—dc21   97–974
                                                    CIP

British Library Cataloguing in Publication Data

A catalogue record for this book is available from the British Library

ISBN 0-471-96225-2

Typeset in 11/13pt Times from the author's disks by Dobbie Typesetting Ltd, Tavistock, Devon
Printed and bound in Great Britain by Bookcraft Ltd, Midsomer Norton
This book is printed on acid-free paper responsibly manufactured from sustainable forestation,
for which at least two trees are planted for each one used for paper production.

Contents

Preface

Immunology for Life Scientists is, as its title suggests, a textbook for students who are studying immunology as part of another degree course. If you consider how we first begin to learn as children, we do so through repeated exposure to words and examples. It is only once we have obtained a working vocabulary and an understanding of what those words mean that we are taught the grammar of the language. Learning a new science may be treated in a similar way. Thus in *Immunology for Life Scientists*, unlike other texts, I have tried to introduce you to immunological terms and concepts (and to explain them fully) using everyday language. I have avoided detailed practical descriptions since, unless you are familiar with the techniques and terminology, they may lead to confusion. This book aims to give students a thorough grounding in the concepts of both basic and clinical immunology and to give them the ability and (I hope) enthusiasm to read review articles and seminal papers which do describe exactly how the work was performed. It is important to learn to walk before you run, and by having a firm grounding and thorough understanding of the concepts of immunology, you should be able to go on to more complex texts without becoming confused or disheartened.

This book is designed as a starting point. For students who wish to learn more or require a fuller understanding of immunology, annotated lists of references and review articles have been included.

Finally, with increasing student numbers there is a move towards self-assessed and self-directed learning. This text is also designed to meet these requirements. It comes with a self-assessment program which can help students to learn and can provide information to tutors about areas of difficulty which may then be addressed in tutorial sessions. Perhaps, most importantly, I hope it will make learning fun!

L.-J. E.

Chapter 1

Cells and Tissues
of the
Immune System

LEARNING OBJECTIVES

In order to understand the way in which the immune system fights infection, it is necessary for you to be able to identify the cells involved and to associate the correct physical (phenotypic) and functional characteristics with them. These attributes (and many other aspects of the immune response) are described using specific terms which have precise meanings. Thus, learning immunology is like learning a new language; once you have mastered the terminology and the basic structure, the rest falls into place quite easily. The cells and tissues of the immune system provide part of the basic structure of immunology, and this chapter places special emphasis on introducing a number of relevant terms which you will come across again and again throughout this book. Thus, the purpose of this chapter is to introduce you to the terminology used to describe the cells involved in the immune response and to describe the physical organisation of the tissues within the body which comprise the immune system.

THE PLURIPOTENT STEM CELL

The **mature cells** of the immune system have a limited lifespan and therefore must be replaced continuously by new ones which arise from **immature precursors**. The latter undergo a series of changes which result in a cell which has the physical characteristics of a mature cell, i.e. which expresses the mature cell **phenotype**. This process is known as **differentiation**.

The precursor cells themselves develop from **progenitor cells** which are thought to have a common origin — the **pluripotent** or **common haemopoietic stem cell** — which is found in the bone marrow. These cells are able to renew themselves by proliferation and can acquire new functional and phenotypic

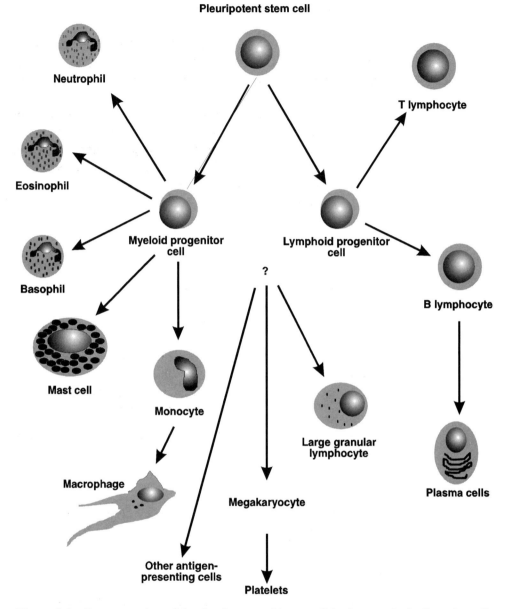

Figure 1.1   Representation of the developmental image of the immunologically active cells

characteristics by differentiating into progenitor cells, e.g. the common erythrocyte, megakaryocyte, myeloid and lymphoid progenitor cells.

The process of blood cell production—**haematopoiesis**—comprises a complex sequence of events (including cell proliferation, differentiation and maturation) that is controlled by a variety of soluble secreted factors (known as **cytokines** and **lymphokines**) and hormones. The developmental lineage of those cells to be described in this chapter is illustrated in Figure 1.1.

The Common Myeloid Progenitor Cell

The common myeloid progenitor cell gives rise to **polymorphonuclear leukocytes** (**PMNs**) which are also known as **granulocytes**. The PMNs are a group of cells which have two major features in common; they have a wide variety (poly) of differently shaped (morpho) nuclei and they all have granules in their cytoplasm. A summary of their characteristics is given in Table 1.1. In addition, the **common myeloid progenitor cell** gives rise to the **monocytes** and **macrophages**. These cells are also known as **mononuclear phagocytes**. They are large (with a diameter of 10–18 µm), have a kidney-shaped nucleus and a relatively large amount of cytoplasm (which may contain very faint, small, **azurophilic** (blue-staining) granules).

The different PMNs may be identified by their staining reactions with Giemsa dye.
a) Neutrophils have blue nuclei, pale blue cytoplasm and small, indistinct, granules.
b) Eosinophils have blue nuclei and red-staining cytoplasmic granules. (Eosin is a red dye.)
c) Basophils have blue nuclei and blue–black cytoplasmic granules.
d) Mast cells have very large blue–black cytoplasmic granules.

Table 1.1 Summary of the characteristics of the polymorphonuclear leukocytes

Name	Characteristics
Polymorphonuclear leukocytes (also known as granulocytes)	Irregularly shaped nuclei; granular cytoplasm
Neutrophils	Pale blue staining, granular cytoplasm; actively phagocytic
Eosinophils	Granular cytoplasm stains red with eosin; slightly phagocytic but most important role is in allergy and resistance to parasitic infections
Basophils	Large, dark blue staining granules; blood-borne; important in allergy; granules contain chemicals which have dramatic effects on muscles and blood vessels
Mast cells	Very large, dark blue staining granules; important in allergy; granules contain chemicals which have dramatic effects on muscles and blood vessels

Neutrophils

Normally, 60–70% of white blood cells are granulocytes and about 90% of these are neutrophils, which provide protection from a variety of micro-organisms and are arguably the most important white blood cells in eliminating non-viral infections. They are relatively large cells (about 10–20 μm in diameter) and, despite their important function, are relatively short-lived (about 2–3 days).

The primary function of these cells is to remove micro-organisms by a process known as **phagocytosis** (a phenomenon which may be compared to the uptake of particulate matter by an amoeba). This involves trapping organisms between 'arms' of cytoplasm — **pseudopodia** — which eventually surround the organism and fuse to form a membrane-bound vesicle within the cell cytoplasm — **the phagosome**. This vesicle fuses with enzyme-containing granules (the **lysosomes**) to form a **phagolysosome** (Figure 1.2). The enzymes released in this way help to kill and break down the trapped organisms, thus participating in the microbicidal activity of the cell.

The granular appearance of these cells is due to the cytoplasmic inclusions they possess. Traditionally, neutrophils have been said to contain two types of granules: **primary** (azurophilic) **granules** (lysosomes), which contain **acid hydrolases**, **myeloperoxidase** and **lysozyme**, and **secondary** (specific) **granules**, which contain lactoferrin and lysozyme but lack myeloperoxidase. However, recently a greater diversity has been observed. It has been suggested that the term specific or secondary granule should be reserved for those peroxidase-negative granules which contain lactoferrin. In addition to the granules, another inclusion has been identified — the secretory vesicle — which acts as an intracellular store of molecules usually found expressed on the cell membrane and which act as receptors for other molecules.

Neutrophils are produced in the bone marrow, whence mature cells pass into the circulation. When appropriate signals occur, neutrophils are activated and emigrate from the blood vessels into the tissues (**chemotaxis**). During this process, they may discharge the contents of their intracellular granules (**degranulation**), which may affect nearby cells or extracellular bacteria and may increase cell-membrane-associated events (such as chemotaxis and the **respiratory burst**) by increased expression of particular membrane proteins. The respiratory burst results in the production of highly reactive chemicals (e.g. reactive oxygen species) which are capable of destroying micro-organisms.

Eosinophils

In healthy people who do not have allergies, 2–5% of the white cells in the blood are **eosinophils**. Like neutrophils, they contain intracellular granules, although those in eosinophils are quite distinct. They are **membrane-bound**

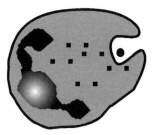
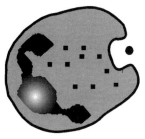

1. Formation of pseudopodia

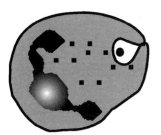
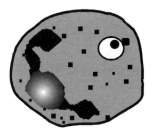

2. Formation of phagosome   **3. Phagosome–lysosome fusion**

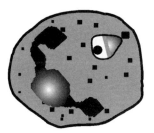
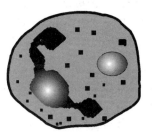

4. Formation of phagolysosome   **5. Destruction of particle**

Figure 1.2   Representation of the process of phagocytosis.
Micro-organisms are removed by phagocytosis, which involves trapping organisms between 'arms' of cytoplasm — pseudopodia — which surround the organism, fusing to form a membrane-bound vesicle — the phagosome. This vesicle fuses with enzyme-containing granules (the lysosomes) to form a phagolysosome. The enzymes released help to kill and break down the trapped organisms

organelles, each with a **crystalline core** that contains four principal cationic proteins which are highly toxic to parasites. Although eosinophils appear to be able to phagocytose, it is not their main function. Parasites such as *Schistosoma mansoni* are too large to phagocytose, so the membranes surrounding the eosinophil granules fuse with the cell membrane and the contents are released outside the eosinophil. The toxic granule proteins help to destroy and eliminate the parasites.

In addition to their anti-parasitic activity, eosinophils have been shown recently to participate in a number of other immunological reactions. They are able to produce a range of soluble factors (cytokines) which may enhance or decrease the cellular functions of a variety of cells (**paracrine action**) or of the producing cell itself (**autocrine action**). Additionally, eosinophils synthesise lipids which stimulate inflammation, a complex series of non-specific reactions which occur in response to tissue damage.

CYTOKINES

These are a group of soluble molecules which are involved in communication between cells. Lymphokines are a group of molecules produced by leukocytes which act as signalling molecules on other cells. All lymphokines are cytokines but not all cytokines are lymphokines.

Basophils and Mast Cells

Basophils comprise less than 0.2% of white blood cells and have many characteristics in common with mast cells. In the past, mast cells have been described as the tissue-based form of the circulating basophil. However, the differentiation pathways of mast cells and basophils are different (Figure 1.3). Basophils leave the bone marrow as mature cells, whilst mast cells leave the bone marrow as precursors and, after migrating to the tissues, proliferate, and differentiate into either **mucosa-associated mast cells** (**MMCs**) or **connective tissue mast cells** (**CTMCs**), depending upon their location.

Basophils and mast cells both play a role in allergic reactions, inflammation, host responses to parasites and cancers, blood vessel generation (**angiogenesis**) and tissue remodelling. Both types of cells have molecules on their surface which allow binding to other cells and to glycoproteins on external surfaces (**surface adhesion receptors**). Recently, it has been suggested that the effects caused by mast cells are mediated, at least in part, through the release of a variety of cytokines.

Murine and human mast cell and basophil lines have been shown to release a range of cytokines, including the interleukins (cytokines produced by white cells which act on white cells) 1, 3, 4, 5, 6, 8, tumour necrosis factor-alpha, granulocyte-macrophage colony-stimulating factor and interferon-gamma.

Mast cell granules are composed of a matrix of proteoglycan (chiefly **heparin**) and neutral proteases (mainly **tryptase**). However, the granules of both

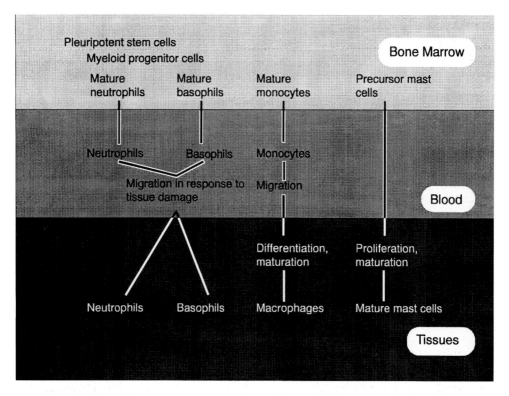

Figure 1.3   Differentiation pathway of basophils and mast cells.
   Basophils leave the bone marrow as mature cells, whilst mast cells leave as precursors. After migrating to the tissues, precursor mast cells proliferate, and differentiate into either mucosa-associated mast cells (MMCs) or connective tissue mast cells (CTMCs)

basophils and mast cells contain **histamine** and other substances which cause the adverse symptoms of allergy and may play a role in immunity to parasites. These include the **slow-releasing substance of anaphylaxis (SRS-A)** and **eosinophil chemotactic factor of anaphylaxis (ECF-A)**. The mechanisms of basophil and mast cell activation and degranulation will be described in a later chapter.

Monocytes and Macrophages

Monocytes circulate in the blood for 1–2 days and migrate to the tissues, where they differentiate into macrophages. Like neutrophils, they are capable of phagocytosis and have lysosomes which contain acid hydrolases and peroxidase, which are important in killing micro-organisms. Despite their having small cytoplasmic granules (lysosomes), these cells are not considered to be granulocytes.

Table 1.2   Tissue macrophages and some of their characteristics

Type	Source	Characteristics
Alveolar macrophages	Lung	Biochemically and functionally distinct subpopulations; lifespan approximately 3 months; may be self-replicating
Kupffer cells	Liver	Subpopulations based on distinct endocytic and lysosomal enzyme activity
Splenic macrophages	Spleen	Subpopulations based on distinct surface antigen expression show distributions in defined areas of the spleen; differences may reflect different functional activity
Microglial cells	Brain	Unknown function; CD4

Macrophages show a range of characteristics which depend on the tissue in which they reside, e.g. **Kupffer cells** of the liver, **microglia cells** of the brain (Table 1.2). This network of related cells is known as the mononuclear phagocyte system (MPS) and used to be referred to as the reticuloendothelial system (RES).

The term mononuclear phagocytes (MPs) includes those cells in the early developmental stages (**monoblasts** and **promonocytes**), monocytes and macrophages. Although true subpopulations of these cells do not exist, macrophages may be categorised according to their stage of development and their state of activation (Table 1.3). In addition to their ability to phagocytose and kill microorganisms, MPs secrete a vast range of chemicals, including clotting factors, complement components and cytokines. They also play an important role in stimulating lymphocyte-specific responses to foreign molecules. This function is known as **antigen presentation**.

Table 1.3   Characterisation of macrophages

Cell type	Description
Resident macrophages	Macrophages which are present in specific sites in normal, non-inflamed tissues
Exudate macrophages	Macrophages found in exudates which are derived from monocytes and share many of their characteristics. Identifiable by peroxidase activity; they are thought to be the precursors of resident macrophages
Elicited macrophages	Macrophages which are attracted to a particular site by a specific stimulus. Elicited macrophages are heterogeneous in both phenotype and function
Activated macrophages	Both resident and elicited macrophages may become activated by appropriate signals (such as the cytokine interferon-gamma). Such cells exhibit increased or new functional activities

The Common Lymphoid Progenitor Cell

The common lymphoid progenitor cell gives rise to **lymphocytes**. These cells, along with monocytes and macrophages, are also known as **mononuclear leukocytes (MNLs)** because, in contrast to the polymorphonuclear leukocytes, they have very regular, spherical to kidney-shaped nuclei.

About 20% of white blood cells are lymphocytes. They are about 6–10 μm in diameter and have a large, almost spherical nucleus surrounded by an indistinct halo of cytoplasm. Their most important characteristic is their ability to specifically recognise foreign molecules such as those of micro-organisms, a feature not possessed by any other cell. This means that any lymphocyte function stimulated by a foreign molecule or **immunogen** is directed solely at that immunogen. Upon stimulation, some lymphocytes become **effector cells**, performing functions designed to eliminate the immunogen, whilst others become long-lived **memory cells**, which may persist for years and allow a more rapid response upon second exposure to the immunogen.

Lymphocytes may be divided into two major populations — **T cells** and **B cells**. Although they are derived from a common progenitor in the bone marrow, they are 'conditioned' by the **thymus** (T cells) or the **bone marrow** (B cells) before they become functionally active.

Early experiments in animals indicated that not only were lymphocytes immunologically active cells but that they were composed of distinct subpopulations. Glick, Chang and Joap (1956) found that by removing the bursa of Fabricius from newborn chicks it was possible to reduce antigen-stimulated antibody production. Later, Aspinall et al (1963) showed that removing the thymus of newborn chicks delayed graft rejection, an effect not seen when the bursa was removed. These experiments suggested the existence of two types of immune response, which became known as cell-mediated and humoral.

These lymphocyte populations may be distinguished by the molecules they express on their surface membrane and by the substances they secrete. T (and other) cells produce lymphokines. By contrast, only B cells produce antibodies. These are globular proteins — **immunoglobulins (Ig)** — which are designed to recognise and bind to specific molecules or groups of molecules known as **antigens**. Antigens which generate an immune response are known as immunogens — this will be covered in greater detail in Chapter 2.

> ## RECEPTORS
>
> Many molecules in the immune system interact with other molecules known as receptors. This ligand–receptor interaction is often likened to the interaction between a lock and key. The key for any particular lock is shaped intricately so that it fits that one lock and no other. However, master keys may fit in many different locks because they share the important common features with the different keys which allow the lock to be opened. Many receptors to which you will be introduced may be considered to be like locks, including the antibody molecules mentioned above. They are designed to recognise a single molecule, a particular antigen—a specific key. However, a different antigen may have the capacity to bind that antibody molecule—a cross-reacting antigen—because it acts like a master key and has the important features of the original antigen.

T and B cell populations can be distinguished by the presence or absence of particular molecules (or markers) on their membranes (Table 1.4). Each population can be divided further into subpopulations based on the presence of particular markers on the cell surface which appear to distinguish groups of cells either with specific functions or at certain stages of development or activation. These markers or molecules have been classified using an internationally recognised system known as the **CD (cluster designation) system** such that molecules are identified as CD1, CD2 etc.

T cells

Originally, human T cells were identified by their ability to bind to sheep red blood cells (SRBCs); this is now known to be due to the presence of the CD2

Table 1.4 Characteristics which distinguish T cells from B cells

Characteristic	T cells	B cells
Cell type	Mononuclear leukocytes	Mononuclear leukocytes
Cell surface molecules which allow the cell to bind antigen the antigen receptor	TCR/CD3	Antibody/BCR
Characteristic surface molecules	CD3, CD4 or CD8	Membrane immunoglobulin, CD19, CD20, CD40
Chief secretory products	Lymphokines	Antibodies

molecule on the T cell surface which acts as a receptor for certain molecules on the surface of the SRBC.

In Bach et al (1969) reported a chance observation that a few human peripheral blood lymphocytes formed clusters (rosettes) when incubated with sheep red blood cells (SRBCs). These clusters comprised a central lymphocyte surrounded by several SRBCs. Several subsequent reports demonstrated that a percentage of human lymphocytes was capable of binding SRBCs. This phenomenon proved to be peculiar to thymus-derived lymphocytes. Rosette formation was shown to occur only with living cells and to be temperature-dependent.

The **T cell antigen receptor (TCR)** is a group of molecules used by T cells to recognise and interact with specific antigen which is presented to them by cells such as macrophages. This receptor associates on the cell surface with a group of membrane-anchored polypeptides known as the **CD3 complex**. Thus, T cells are now identified by the expression of CD3. Furthermore, they may be subdivided according to the presence or absence of other surface molecules. Thus, in the blood, some T cells express the CD4 molecule whilst a distinct set express the CD8 molecule. Previously, these molecules were thought to define functionally distinct subsets of T cells. CD4+ T cells were known as **helper cells** (e.g. they helped B cells to produce antibody) and CD8+ T cells as **cytotoxic cells** (they were capable of killing certain cells). This division is becoming less obvious, since some CD4+ cells may have cytotoxic activity.

T helper cells in mice have been subdivided according to the lymphokines they produce. These subsets have been designated **Th0, Th1** and **Th2** cells. In general, Th1 cells produce lymphokines which stimulate macrophages and cytotoxic T cells, Th2 cells produce lymphokines which stimulate B cells to proliferate and produce antibody, whilst Th0 cells produce a mixture of lymphokines and are thought to be an intermediate stage from which Th1 and Th2 cells are derived (Figure 1.4). In humans, Th1- and Th2-like cells have been demonstrated, although they do not seem to show the strict division seen in mice with respect to their patterns of cytokine secretion. Recently, similar subsets have been proposed for CD8+ T cells.

B cells

B cells comprise about 5–15% of circulating lymphocytes. A distinguishing feature of B cells is the expression of antibody molecules (immunoglobulin) on their surface (**mIg**) which act as the antigen receptor for the cell. Like that expressed on T lymphocytes, the B cell antigen receptor (**BCR**) consists of more

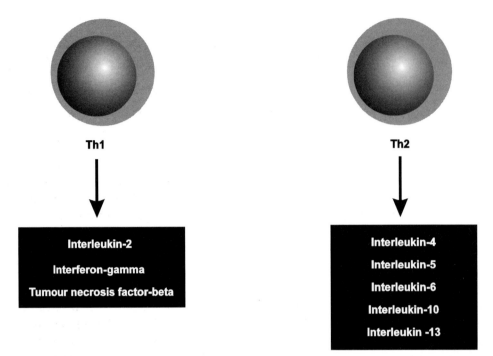

Figure 1.4   Th subpopulations and some of the cytokines they produce.

   T helper cells in mice have been subdivided according to the lymphokines they produce. These subsets have been designated Th0, Th1 and Th2 cells. In general, Th1 cells produce lymphokines which stimulate macrophages and cytotoxic T cells, whilst Th2 cells produce lymphokines which stimulate B cells to proliferate and produce antibody. In humans, Th1- and Th2-like cells do not seem to show the strict cytokine secretion patterns seen in mice

than one group of molecules. In addition to mIg, the BCR comprises a duplex of molecules known as Igα and Igβ which have a single extracellular domain and a cytoplasmic tail. The detailed structure of both the T and B cell antigen receptors will be discussed in Chapter 3.

   Each antibody molecule contains a region which recognises and binds to a particular antigen. The genetic code for this region within B cells is highly variable, allowing the antibody coded for by each cell to recognise a distinct antigen. However, all the antibody molecules coded for by a single cell have the same amino acid sequence and recognise the same antigen. The progeny of a B cell (the new cells produced when a B cell divides) all have the code for antibody which recognises the same antigen as the parent cell. However, owing to

The fact that the progeny of a single B cell all produce antibody of the same specificity was exploited in the 1960s to produce a tool which is widely used in many different scientific disciplines. B cells which had been stimulated by immunogen were mixed with tumour cells derived from B lymphocytes which grow indefinitely but do not produce antibody. By using a chemical to fuse the different cells, the resulting product was a B cell which grew indefinitely and produced antibody of the same specificity as the original B cell. This meant that an endless supply of highly specific, monoclonal antibody could be produced to virtually any immunogen. Such monoclonal antibodies have allowed us to identify molecules on the surface of cells, to quantify both antibody and antigen, and are used in numerous immunological techniques.

various influences during B cell mitosis, the variable sequence of the antibody produced by the daughter cells may be slightly different to that of the parent cell. Usually, this does not alter which antigen the antibody recognises, but it may alter the strength of attraction between the antibody and its antigen.

Pre-B cells are derived from the common lymphoid progenitor. They are large and have parts of antibody molecules in their cytoplasm. They differentiate into immature and then mature B cells which have antibody and other molecules on their membranes (e.g. CD19, CD20, CD23, CD24, CD35 and CD40). After exposure to an antigen (antigenic stimulation or challenge), B cells proliferate and differentiate either into plasma cells or small, resting cells which are able to respond the next time that the same antigen is encountered (memory cells). Plasma cells are designed to manufacture vast quantities of antibody which is secreted outside the cell. Since the plasma cells inherit the genetic code of their parental cell, the specificity of the secreted antibody will be the same as that expressed on the surface of the parental cell.

Large Granular Lymphocytes

Large granular lymphocytes (LGLs; also known as third population cells, null cells, non-T, non-B cells) are a group which, in general, 'look like' lymphocytes but which lack the major, definitive, markers of either T or B cells (TCR and mIg) and have distinctly granular cytoplasm. These cells account for 20% of blood lymphocytes and the markers that they do express are usually found on T cells or cells of the mononuclear phagocyte system. It is unclear whether these cells are derived from the common lymphocyte progenitor or from another cell which, as yet, has not been identified.

Table 1.5 Characteristics of large granular lymphocytes

Characteristic	NK cells	Killer cells	LAK cells
Other cell types performing function	None	Macrophages/PMN	None
Mechanism involved in killing	Pore-forming proteins	Antibody-mediated lysis	Pore-forming proteins
Target cells	Some tumour cells; virally infected cells	Antibody-sensitised cells	All tumour cells
MHC restriction	None	None	None

Amongst the large granular lymphocytes are a number of cells with distinct functional activity (Table 1.5). These include the **natural killer cells (NK cells)**, the **killer cells (K cells)** and the **lymphokine-activated killer cells (LAK cells)**.

1. Natural killer cells can kill certain tumour cells and some virally infected cells, but unlike cytotoxic T cells they are not capable of recognising a specific antigen. However, they show some selectivity in their actions, being able to bind to and kill only a limited range of cells (their target cells).
2. Killer cells (K cells) have molecules on their surface which act as receptors for the end of an antibody molecule which does not bind antigen, i.e. the **Fc region** of the molecule.

THE ANTIBODY MOLECULE

This consists of three major functional regions called the $F(ab)_2$ region, the hinge region and the Fc region. The $F(ab)_2$ region (fragment antigen binding) contains the antigen-binding sites of the molecule, the Fc region (fragment crystallisable) confers the biological properties of the molecule and the hinge region is where the other two meet and confers flexibility on the molecule.

Using these Fc receptors, K cells are able to bind to cells which have antibody attached to them via their antigen-binding regions and kill them. Thus, if a cell is infected with a virus and some of the viral proteins are present in the cell membrane, antibodies formed against them will bind to the viral antigens on the surface of the cell. A killer cell can bind to this antibody, is thereby activated and kills the virally infected (target) cell. This activity is known as **antibody-dependent cellular cytotoxicity (ADCC)** and may be performed by some cytotoxic T cells as well (Figure 1.5).

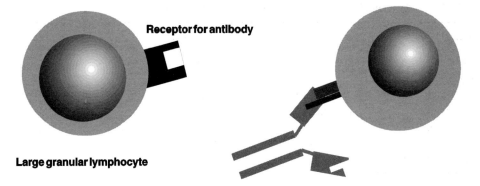

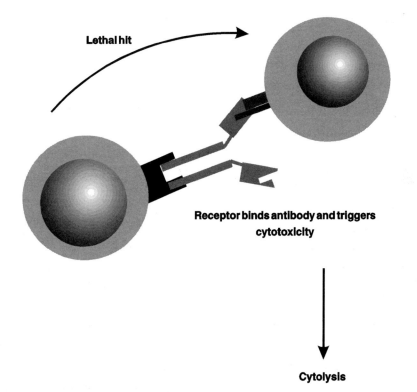

Figure 1.5 Antibody-dependent cellular cytotoxicity.

In a virally infected cell, some of the viral proteins are expressed on the cell membrane, allowing virus-specific antibodies to bind to them. A killer cell can attach to this antibody using its Fc receptor and is thereby activated and kills the virally infected target cell. This activity is known as antibody-dependent cellular cytotoxicity (ADCC)

3. Lymphokine-activated killer cells can be produced in vitro by incubating mononuclear cells with the lymphokine, **interleukin-2**. Like NK cells, LAK cells do not specifically recognise an antigen but they are capable of destroying a wider range of targets than NK cells. LAK cells may be derived from NK cells or cytotoxic T cells.

Dendritic Cells

Dendritic cells are irregularly shaped and actively extrude and retract thread-like 'fingers' of cytoplasm and surrounding cell membrane. They are found in most tissues of the body but their stage of maturation may vary with their location. These specialised cells, which play a critical role in initiating immune responses, may transport antigen within them or on their surface and thus, like macrophages, play an important role in helping T cells to respond to antigen. However, unlike macrophages, they are non-phagocytic (in culture) and may be only weakly adherent.

Cells resembling dendritic cells have been found in the fluid which drains from the tissues — the lymph. These **veiled cells** may be derived from tissue-based dendritic cells such as **Langerhans cells** of the skin.

Megakaryocytes and Platelets

Megakaryocytic progenitor cells are derived from haematopoietic stem cells. They undergo **endomitosis** (producing multiple copies of DNA within the cell) and differentiate into megakaryocytes. Thus, mature megakaryocytes are large, polyploid cells with distinct, folded membranes. A pool is maintained in the bone marrow to replenish stocks in the blood when required. This may be controlled by the lymphokine IL-3, a potent stimulator of megakaryocyte progenitor cells. Megakaryocytes give rise to platelets by a process which appears to involve cytoplasmic fragmentation of the cell. Platelet production depends on the number and size of megakaryocytes in the marrow and is stimulated by **thrombopoietin**.

In recent years, the immunological relevance of platelets has become fully established. It is now clear that these cells possess granules containing a variety of substances which affect the clotting and immune systems. A major constituent of platelet **alpha granules** is **thrombospondin**, which plays an important role in blood coagulation. Also, **platelet-derived endothelial cell growth factor** (**PD-ECGF**) stimulates the growth and directed movement (**chemotaxis**) of endothelial cells in vitro and angiogenesis in vivo.

TISSUES OF THE IMMUNE SYSTEM

Although lymphocytes are found circulating in the blood, a large proportion of them are found either in discrete clusters or organised in specific tissues. This distribution increases the chance of an antigen meeting a cell which bears a receptor capable of binding it. The components of this **lymphoid system** may

Imagine arranging to meet a friend in a busy shopping mall. If you did not state a precise meeting point the likelihood of the two of you meeting amongst the crowd would be very remote. However, arranging to meet at a particular place would ensure that you would meet, provided you waited long enough for your friend to arrive. This is the logic behind the organisation of lymphoid tissue. Antigen-specific cells are located in a tissue through which any foreign molecules will eventually drain, thus increasing the likelihood of the cells meeting their specific antigen.

be categorised as **primary**, **secondary** or **tertiary lymphoid tissue**. Primary lymphoid tissues are involved in the development and differentiation of T and B lymphocytes and include the thymus and the bursa equivalent tissues (which are the fetal liver and, probably, the adult bone marrow respectively, in humans).

Glick, Chang and Joap (1956) performed a series of experiments using newborn chicks. In some birds they removed a small organ near the cloaca (equivalent of the mammalian anus) called the bursa. When challenged with antigen, these chicks were unable to produce specific antibody, which led the authors to conclude that, in chickens, B cells develop in the bursa of Fabricius.

They are responsible for the production of mature 'virgin' lymphocytes, i.e. those which have not yet been exposed to antigen. Secondary lymphoid tissues are designed to allow the accumulation and presentation of antigen to both virgin and memory lymphocyte populations. The remainder of the body's tissues may be considered 'tertiary' lymphoid tissues, in that they normally contain only a few lymphocytes, but, during an inflammatory reaction, may be invaded by unique subsets of memory lymphocytes.

The lymphoid tissues are further subdivided into discrete microenvironments, each characterised by a distinct complement of lymphocyte subsets and **stromal** cells (non-specialised cells which form the skeleton of the tissue or organ). This distribution arises as a result of **lymphocyte homing**, a phenomenon whereby lymphocytes seek out and localise to specific microenvironments in response to a number of physiological processes. These homing mechanisms play a vital role in the distribution of naive and memory lymphocytes that are required for effective **immune surveillance**.

The Thymus

During development, the thymus is the first organ to produce lymphocytes and provides an environment for T cell maturation. It has two lobes divided by **trabeculae** (or connective tissue 'walls') into **lobules**, each of which has an outer **cortex** and an inner **medulla**. The thymic epithelium is thought to secrete a factor which attracts **thymocytes** (immature, pre-T cells) to the thymus. These cells differentiate into **mature T cells** as they pass from the cortex to the medulla, whence they are released to populate the peripheral lymphoid tissue.

Approximately three-quarters of all the lymphocytes in the thymus are located in the deeper cortex. These cells express CD1 and both CD4 and CD8 (T cells in the blood express either CD4 or CD8). As the cells pass into the medulla, they lose either CD4 or CD8 expression, reflecting genetic rearrangement which may cause the death of the cell. Indeed, the majority of cells produced in the thymus die there. A portion of the cells that are inactivated by the thymus are those which might otherwise cause damage to normal body cells (**autoimmune T cells**).

Thymic lymphocytes are surrounded by epithelial cells and other supporting cells, including interdigitating reticular cells and macrophages. In the cortex, supporting cells include the **thymic nurse cells**, whose function is unknown but which appear to contain thymocytes. It has been suggested that the nurse cells may influence the development of thymocytes. In the medulla, and at the junction between the cortex and medulla where most blood vessels are situated, there are interdigitating cells which are derived from the bone marrow and are a type of dendritic cell.

The epithelial cells of the thymus produce a number of hormones, including **thymulin, thymosin α1, thymosin β4**, and **thymopoietin**, which are required for the differentiation of thymic precursors into mature cells. The characteristic **Hassal's corpuscles** which are found within the medulla of the thymus are concentric agglomerations of epithelial cells.

Bursa of Fabricius and Mammalian 'Bursa Equivalents'

The bursa of Fabricius in birds is a lymphoepithelial organ located near the cloaca. Birds which have this organ removed are not able to mount a normal antibody response when stimulated with an antigen. Thus, the bursa is a primary lymphoid tissue in mammals concerned with the development and differentiation of B cells. In mammals, those tissues which most closely resemble the bursa include the gut-associated lymphoid tissues (including the appendix and Peyer's patches), the fetal liver and, following birth, the bone marrow.

The Lymphatic System

Within the body there are two circulatory systems, the blood and the lymph. Blood flows around the body through a complex of arteries, veins and capillaries. Components of the blood which leave the vessels and enter the tissues comprise the extracellular fluid. This fluid returns to the blood by draining into a network of vessels called lymphatics. At the junction between major lymph vessels are found small, bean-shaped, discrete aggregates of tissue called **lymph nodes**. Several vessels may bring the lymph to a particular node (afferent lymphatics) and usually a single vessel (the efferent lymphatic) carries it away. The lymph carries antigen from the tissues to the lymph nodes, where immune responses are initiated.

Lymphocytes can enter the lymphatic circulation directly from the blood, to which they return via the **thoracic duct**—a lymphatic vessel draining into the circulation close to the heart. This traffic of lymphocytes is known as **recirculation** (Figure 1.6) and occurs at specialised sites called high endothelial venules (HEVs), found particularly in lymph nodes and the Peyer's patches (collections of lymphoid tissue in the gut). HEVs are blood vessels in which the endothelial cells that line them have a high columnar structure which is distinct to that in other areas. However, the presence of HEVs and even lymph nodes is not essential for lymphocyte recirculation.

Leukocytes have special membrane molecules called homing receptors which allow them to bind to particular HEVs and other endothelia. As a result, lymphocytes adhere to the walls of vessels in a process called **margination**, and then pass between the cells of the blood vessels in a process called **diapedesis** into the surrounding tissues, from whence they return via the lymph back to the blood.

The movement or **traffic** of cells through the body to certain areas is called **migration**. When splenic T cells are re-injected into the blood, a large number of the cells return to this organ rather than to other sites. This directed migration of cells to particular tissue sites is called **homing**.

Lymph Nodes

The lymph nodes are bean-shaped structures usually found at the junction between major lymphatic vessels. They range between 1 and 25 mm in diameter but become much larger during an infection. A normal, resting lymph node has three main areas, the cortex, the paracortical areas and the medulla. It is

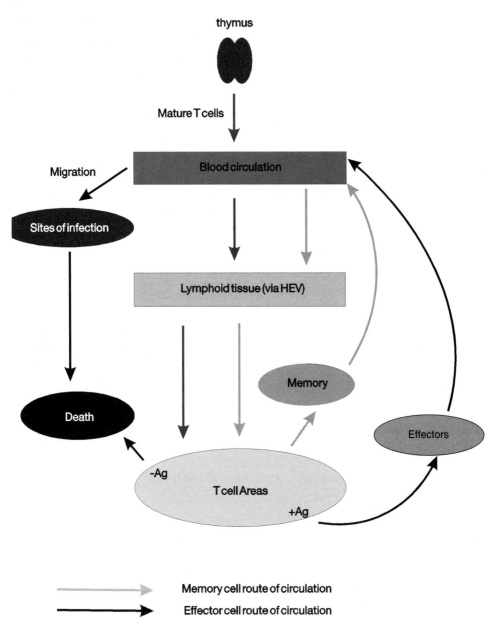

Figure 1.6   Lymphocyte recirculation.

Lymphocytes can enter the lymphatic circulation directly from the blood, to which they return via the thoracic duct. This traffic of lymphocytes is known as recirculation and occurs at specialised sites called high endothelial venules. Leukocytes have special receptors called homing receptors which allow them to bind to the walls of blood vessels at these sites and pass into the tissues, whence they return, via the lymph, back to the blood

surrounded by a capsule and the cells within it are supported by a fine meshwork known as a reticulum. Lymph (in the afferent lymphatic vessels) comes into the lymph node at the subcapsular sinus. In addition, lymph nodes have a blood supply and lymphocytes may enter the node directly from the blood through HEVs in the paracortex. The flow of cells is towards the medulla at the centre (centripetal), where they drain into the major efferent lymphatic duct in the hilus of the node to be conducted away.

Once in the lymph node, lymphocytes locate according to type such that T lymphocytes tend to collect in the paracortical areas and B cells go to the outer edge of the cortex. This pattern of distribution may be affected by other cells in these areas, e.g. interdigitating cells in the T cell areas and follicular dendritic cells (FDCs) in the B-dependent areas. The paracortical region contains large lymphocytes and blast-like cells and is easily distinguished from the cortex. Also, the medulla contains numerous plasma cells which actively secrete antibody.

Typical T and B lymphocytes in the secondary lymphoid organs are long-lived cells that are selected from a large pool of short-lived precursor cells in the primary lymphoid organs. The bulk of mature T and B cells are immunologically naive and remain inactive for long periods of time. Contact with specific antigen causes these cells to proliferate rapidly and differentiate into a mixture of short-lived effector cells and long-lived memory cells. Survival of memory cells appears to require persistent contact with antigen.

The B cells form dense aggregates which are known as follicles. **Primary follicles** are very dense and uniform, and their centres may contain some larger cells often associated with macrophages. This zone is known as the **germinal centre**. Following exposure to antigen, the lymph node shows an increased turnover of lymphocytes. The follicles of the cortex become much larger, with prominent germinal centres composed of metabolically active and mitotic cells and are known as **secondary follicles**.

Germinal Centres

The B cells that give rise to germinal centres have to be activated outside the follicles in the T cell-rich zones (Figure 1.7). After a single immunisation of a protein antigen, oligoclonal germinal centres form, each of which comprises usually three B cell blasts which undergo clonal expansion (replication) and site-directed hypermutation of immunoglobulin-variable (Ig-v) region genes. Mature germinal centres are divided into dark and light zones. The proliferating blasts, **centroblasts**, occupy the dark zone and give rise to **centrocytes** that fill the light zone which contains FDCs capable of taking up antigen and expressing it on their surface for more than a year.

Germinal centres last for about 3 weeks following immunisation. After subsequent exposure to the same antigen, they reappear but their size decreases

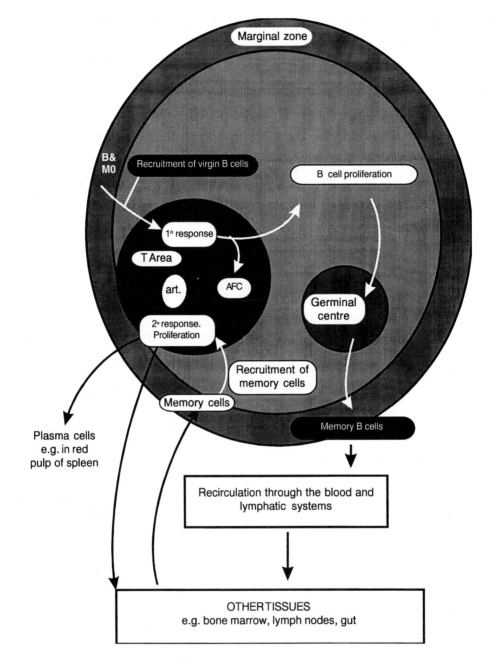

Figure 1.7 Cellular distribution in lymphoid follicles.

B cells that give rise to germinal centres are activated outside the follicles in T-cell-rich zones. Mature germinal centres consist of dark and light zones. The proliferating centroblasts occupy the dark zone and give rise to centrocytes that fill the light zone, which contains follicular dendritic cells (FDCs) capable of taking up antigen and expressing it on their surface. art. = arteriole; AFC = antibody-forming cell; Mo = macrophage

with successive immunisations. In the next few months, follicular memory B blasts continue to proliferate. These cells probably provide the source of plasma and memory cells needed to maintain antibody production and memory.

Primary Follicles

When follicles are not involved in antigen responses, the principal cellular components are recirculating B cells passing through a network of follicular dendritic cells. Although the main lymphocyte type in the primary follicles of lymph nodes is the naive, recirculating B cell, in splenic follicles there are also some mature, non-recirculating B cells.

Spleen

The spleen is a secondary lymphoid organ but also performs several other non-immunological functions. Like the lymph nodes, it has a capsule with fibrous partitions (septae) that penetrate the body of the spleen. There are two main types of tissue, the white and red pulp. The erythroid red pulp serves as a filter for damaged or aged red cells. Lymphocytes enter and leave the spleen predominantly via the bloodstream.

The white pulp consists of cells and tissues surrounding the major arterial branches — the periarteriolar sheath (PALS) — and associated clusters of lymphocytes — the lymphatic follicles or nodules. These follicles have a similar cellular arrangement as those described in lymph nodes. Thus, the B cell-dependent area of the spleen consists of the lymphoid follicles and the T cell-dependent area consists of the PALS.

The histological changes seen in the spleen after antigenic stimulation are similar to those described in the lymph nodes, with the development of distinct germinal centres in the secondary follicles.

Mucosa-associated Lymphoid Tissue

This term is used to describe the diffusely distributed lymphoid tissues in the linings (mucosa) of the gastrointestinal, respiratory and urogenital tracts. However, the gut-associated lymphoid tissue (GALT) and the bronchus-associated lymphoid tissue (BALT) are the best characterised.

GALT is made up of Peyer's patches and isolated follicles in the tissue beneath the mucosa of the colon (colonic submucosa). Lymphocytes are also found in the lamina propria, the intestinal epithelium and the lumen of the intestine. Peyer's patches are aggregates of lymphocytes where the B cells form a central follicle and are surrounded by T cells and macrophages which help T cells to recognise antigen (i.e. they act as antigen-presenting cells). These patches have efferent lymphatics that drain into mesenteric lymph nodes, but no afferent lymphatics. They are covered by a specialised lymphoepithelium consisting of mucosa-associated lymphoid or M cells. Antigens in the gut can enter the Peyer's patches via the M cells, which selectively take up particles. It is not known whether these cells actually change (process) the antigens in any way or merely deliver them to the lymphoid follicles.

BALT is structurally similar to GALT. It consists of large collections of lymphocytes (the majority of which are B cells), organised into aggregates and follicles with few germinal centres. These are found primarily along the main bronchi in the lungs. The epithelium covering BALT follicles lacks goblet cells and cilia. M cells which cover the BALT follicles are structurally similar to intestinal M cells. BALT contains an elaborate network of capillaries, arterioles and venules, and efferent lymphatics. This suggests that BALT may play a role in sampling antigen not only from the lungs but also from the systemic circulation.

LEARNING OUTCOMES

Having studied this chapter you should now have a basic knowledge of the principal cells and tissues involved in the immune response. This should include an understanding of the physical and functional characteristics of the cells and how to distinguish between them. You should also have a mental picture of the tissue environment in which immune responses normally occur. You may supplement this basic information by reading the material suggested in Further Reading. Since understanding immunology requires you to effectively learn a 'new language' it is important to ensure that you understand the meaning of the terms used and that you remember them whilst you progress through the subject. To help with this, test yourself on Chapter 1 using the program which accompanies this text. This will help you to assess how well you have understood the material and will help you to remember what you have learnt when you progress to the next chapter. Some of the questions may be based on information available in the Further Reading material.

Chapter 2

Immunogens and Immunogenicity

LEARNING OBJECTIVES

An important characteristic of the immune system is that the cells are able to distinguish between those molecules that are normally present in the body and those that are not. This recognition of 'self' and 'non-self' is a vital distinction. The term 'non-self' may mean a foreign invader such as a micro-organism or a protein expressed on a cell in an abnormal way. Certain areas of the body are known as immunologically privileged sites and are not routinely exposed to immunologically active cells, e.g. the brain. The molecules expressed by cells in these areas may not be expressed elsewhere in the body. If a breach occurs allowing immune cells into these sites, they may attack the tissue because they do not recognise the characteristic molecules of this tissue as self.

This chapter is designed to introduce you to the terms used to describe those substances which stimulate an immune response—**immunogens**. It will discuss those characteristics which make a molecule a good immunogen and will distinguish between an immunogen and an **antigen**—a molecule or group of molecules which bind specific receptors but may not alone induce an immune response. We will also look at one important group of molecules—the **major histocompatibility antigens**.

CHARACTERISTICS OF ANTIGENS AND IMMUNOGENS

An immunogen is any molecule or group of molecules which can induce an immune response, whilst an antigen is any substance which can react with antigen-specific receptors such as membrane immunoglobulin on B cells and the antigen receptor on T cells. Thus, an antigen differs from an immunogen because, although an antigen can interact in a specific way with the immune system, it cannot by itself stimulate an immune response; other stimuli are required. Thus, **all immunogens are antigens but not all antigens are immunogens**.

Lymphocytes possess receptors which bind specific antigens. The antigen receptor on B cells is immunoglobulin, which is anchored in the cell membrane. That on T cells is known as the T cell antigen receptor (TCR). That part of an antigen which binds to these receptors is known as the **antigenic determinant** or **epitope**. An antigen may be protein, lipid, carbohydrate or any combination of these. It may be soluble or particulate, simple or complex, and have many different antigenic determinants (for example, a bacterium may have antigenic determinants on the cell wall, the flagellum or on pili). Although an antigen may have many different antigenic determinants, each of which comprises a small number of amino acids (4–6) or sugar residues, the resulting immune response may result in the production of antibodies which recognise only a few of these. The epitopes recognised may be quite different in two individuals, suggesting that the range of epitopes recognised is under genetic control.

FACTORS AFFECTING IMMUNOGENICITY

A number of physical and biochemical characteristics determine the immunogenicity of a substance. These will be considered below.

Foreignness

The immune system is designed to eliminate anything which does not belong in the normal healthy body, i.e. it is capable of distinguishing between self and non-self; it can recognise things that are foreign to it. Thus, the more foreign a molecule is, the more likely it is that the immune system will react to it and the more immunogenic it will be. It is important to remember that a molecule may not be immunogenic in the host where it is normally found, but may become so if introduced into a different host. For example, rabbit serum albumin injected into a rabbit will not be immunogenic. The same molecule injected into a cow will stimulate an immune response. Also, antibodies are glycoproteins and when injected into a different host (e.g. rabbit antibody into mice) they are immunogenic (because they are complex, foreign proteins).

Size

The size of a molecule appears to affect its immunogenicity. Generally, substances with molecular masses greater than 100 kDa are potent immunogens, whilst those with molecular masses of less than 10 kDa may not stimulate an immune response at all.

Although some small molecules may contain antigenic determinants, i.e. have epitopes capable of binding to antigen receptors on T and B lymphocytes, they are not large enough to stimulate an effective immune response. However, these molecules may be made immunogenic by attaching them to a larger molecule known as a **carrier**. Under these circumstances, the small antigenic molecule is known as a **hapten**.

Chemical Complexity

The chemical complexity of a molecule may affect its ability to stimulate an immune response. Large polymers of amino acids might be expected to be good immunogens (because of their size) but only prove to be so when they consist of a mixture of amino acids.

The types of amino acids present in a peptide also affect its immunogenicity. The presence of aromatic amino acids in a molecule makes it more immunogenic than non-aromatic molecules. This is because the interaction between an antigen and its specific receptor on lymphocytes is governed by non-covalent, hydrophobic forces.

Route of Administration

The type of immune response elicited by an immunogen may be very different at one particular site in the body compared to another. Thus, the route by which an antigen gains access to the immune system may affect its immunogenicity. For example, an organism which normally causes infection when introduced into the lungs (a respiratory pathogen) may be destroyed by the acid in the gut if swallowed.

Dose

The dose of an antigen also may affect its ability to be immunogenic. If it is given at too high or too low a dose, the immune system may fail to respond to an antigen which at the correct dose is immunogenic.

Host Genetic Make-up

Since the magnitude of an elicited immune response reflects the immunogenicity of a molecule, and an individual's ability to mount an immune response is genetically controlled, the genetic make-up of the host must play a role in determining the relative immunogenicity of that molecule. This is exemplified by the fact that some antigens which stimulate an immune response in humans

Table 2.1   Factors affecting the immunogenicity of a molecule

Factor	Explanation
Size	Large molecules are better than small (> 100 kDa)
Foreignness	The more foreign a molecule, the better an immunogen it is
Complexity	Heterogeneous amino acid composition improves immunogenicity
Amino acid type	Aromatic amino acids make a molecule more immunogenic
Route of administration	Immunogenicity may be affected by route of administration; for example, respiratory tract pathogens may be destroyed in the gut
Dose of antigen	Too high or too low a dose fails to stimulate a response and may prevent response on subsequent exposure
Genetic make-up of host	The generation of an immune response is under genetic control

are non-immunogenic in other animals. All the factors affecting the immunogenicity of a molecule are summarised in Table 2.1.

Approaches Used to Increase Immunogenicity

One of the aims of an immune response is to eliminate whatever has stimulated it, e.g. a micro-organism. Obviously, in the case of infection, elimination must be quick and effective to prevent extensive damage to the host (**pathology**). However, where an immunogen is introduced specifically to stimulate a long-lasting immunity (e.g. in the case of immunisation), the longer it is present, the stronger and more long-lasting the resulting immune response will be. This **persistence** can be achieved by mixing the immunogen with an **adjuvant**. There are a number of adjuvants which are commonly used, and whilst their precise method of action is not known exactly, they all increase the strength and longevity of an immune response to a particular immunogen. It is thought that this effect may be achieved in one or more of the following ways: increasing the effective size of the immunogen; enhancing persistence of the immunogen; activating cells such as macrophages and lymphocytes.

THYMUS-DEPENDENT AND
-INDEPENDENT ANTIGENS

When B lymphocytes produce antibody in response to an immunogen, they usually require help from T lymphocytes in the form of soluble factors—**lymphokines**. Immunogens which require such T cell help are known as **T-dependent**. However, a few molecules can stimulate antibody production without T cell help. These are usually large molecules made up of repeating subunits, e.g. bacterial polysaccharides. These **T-independent** immunogens have several copies of each subunit and thus have many copies of each epitope. It is thought that this allows the immunogen to simultaneously link together several antigen receptors on the surface of a single cell. This delivers a large enough stimulus to the cell to cause its activation. However, not all molecules which have a repeating subunit structure are T-independent immunogens. If the basic unit is simple and lacking in complexity, the molecule may not be immunogenic or may require T cell help, e.g. poly-L-lysine.

T-independent antigens usually stimulate the formation of a type of antibody known as IgM. This is probably because the majority of B cells have IgM as their surface antigen receptor. Also, these antigens rarely induce the formation of B memory cells — which cause the rapid development of a highly specific response upon subsequent exposure to the antigen.

ANTIGEN RECOGNITION BY LYMPHOCYTES

Both T and B lymphocytes have receptors on their surface which recognise specific antigen. However, these receptors perform their function in different ways.

B lymphocytes may bind antigen in solution or suspension and recognise the **three-dimensional conformation** of an epitope. In a protein antigen, the conformation of an epitope is affected by the sequence and type of amino acids present. The attractive and repulsive charges associated with each amino acid affect the way in which a protein molecule folds. Thus, a change in the amino acids within a B cell epitope may affect its ability to bind to the B cell antigen receptor, depending on how radical is the change (e.g. a hydrophobic for a hydrophilic, or a charged for a non-charged amino acid) and whether the particular amino acid is directly involved in the binding of the epitope to the receptor.

In contrast to B cells, T lymphocytes bind **linear arrays** of approximately nine amino acids. These cells cannot directly bind antigen; it must be broken down to its primary structure (processed) and presented to the T lymphocyte in association with certain molecules on the surface of antigen-presenting cells (such as macrophages and dendritic cells).

Thus, B cell antigen receptors can recognise epitopes on the surface of complex antigens whilst T cell antigen receptors can recognise epitopes exposed when the molecule is broken down (Figure 2.1).

The molecules on the surface of the antigen-presenting cells which are required for the recognition of antigen by T cells are part of a group of molecules known as the **human leukocyte antigens (HLAs)**. These are coded for by a group of genes known as the **major histocompatibility complex (MHC)**.

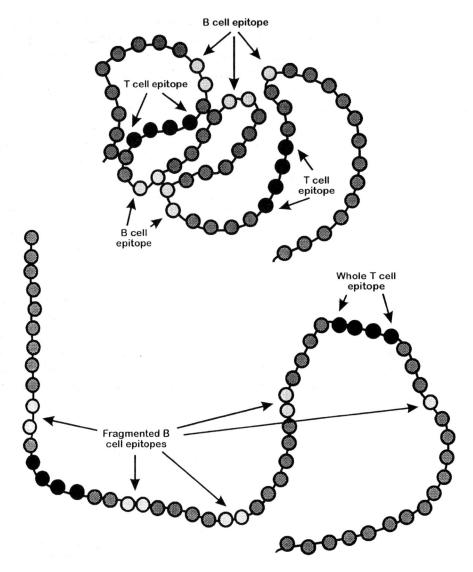

Figure 2.1 B and T cell epitopes.

B cell antigen receptors recognise the three-dimensional conformation of epitopes, whilst T cells recognise linear ones. Thus B cells recognise epitopes on the surface of complex antigens, whilst T cell antigen receptors recognise those exposed when the molecule is broken down

THE MAJOR HISTOCOMPATIBILITY COMPLEX

Molecules expressed on cell surface membranes may act as antigens when introduced to a foreign host. Probably the best examples of this are the blood group antigens A, B and O. An individual of blood group A will have erythrocytes which express this antigen, and if an A+ individual is given group B blood (which expresses the B antigen), the recipient's immune system will recognise the B antigen as foreign and will cause the clumping and destruction of the transfused blood. For this reason, blood must be matched for transfusion. All other cells of the body express a variety of molecules, the natures of which are determined by the genetic make-up of the host. These **tissue antigens** are quite distinct in each individual, and when an organ is transplanted, the donor must be matched to the recipient. If the tissues are not matched, the recipient's immune system will recognise the donor tissue antigens as foreign and will destroy the transplant.

It has long been known that if a mouse is grafted with skin from a genetically distinct mouse, it will reject the graft. By contrast, if the graft is from a genetically identical mouse, the graft survives and is accepted. These early observations led to the discovery of the human leukocyte antigens (HLAs). These are a group of molecules expressed on the surface of cells which, when the cells are introduced to a genetically distinct individual, act as immunogens and stimulate an immune response. It is these molecules which are identified when an individual is 'tissue-typed'. These molecules are products of a group of genes known as the major histocompatibility complex (MHC) in humans. The MHC comprises a large number of separate genes which occupy about 1/3000th of the total genome (Figure 2.2). The genes are divided into three classes. Class I includes the A, B and C region genes, Class II includes the D region genes and

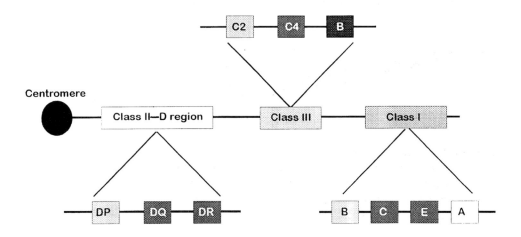

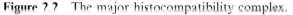

Figure 2.2   The major histocompatibility complex.
The MHC comprises a large number of separate genes which, in humans, occupy about 1/3000th of the total genome. The genes are divided into three classes: Class 1 includes the A, B and C region genes; Class 2 includes the D region genes; Class 3 includes those which produce some of the enzymes and control elements which form part of a group of serum proteins known as complement

Class III includes those genes which produce some of the enzymes and control elements forming part of a group of serum proteins known as complement (see Chapter 7).

Class I MHC Molecules

Antigens coded for by the MHC Class I genes are found on the surface of all nucleated cells and platelets. These are the antigens which are 'typed' when an individual needs an organ transplant. The antigenically distinct molecules are coded for by different regions within the Class I genome (on chromosome 6). These regions are known as A, B and C, and the molecules coded for by these regions are classed as A1, A2, B1, B2 etc.

Structure of Class I Molecules

Class I molecules have one glycosylated polypeptide chain encoded for by the MHC (Figure 2.3). This chain has a molecular mass of 45 kDa and is anchored through the cell membrane. It is non-covalently linked with another molecule — β_2-microglobulin (12 kDa) — which is not coded for by the MHC and is not membrane bound. The heavy or α chain has five distinct regions or **domains**, three of which are extracellular and hydrophilic (the α1, α2 and α3 globular domains), one of which is transmembraneous and hydrophobic and one of which is cytoplasmic and hydrophilic. This molecule is similar in structure to antibody and the genes which code for the MHC Class I antigens are considered to be part of the **immunoglobulin supergene family**. The majority of the differences which distinguish the Class I antigens from each other (i.e. the antigenic determinants) result from amino acid differences in the α1 and α2 domains. In addition, a number of antigenically distinct versions of the same molecule (known as **polymorphism**) may be seen.

β_2-microglobulin is a polypeptide chain with a single domain which is structurally similar to MHC (and immunoglobulin) domains. This molecule plays a vital role in transporting newly synthesised MHC proteins to the cell surface.

Class I molecules present antigen to those T cells which have the CD8 molecule on their surface (most cytotoxic T cells). This ability to present antigen is related to the structure of the molecule. Each of the α1 and α2 domains consists of four β strands and an α helix. Together these β strands form a β-pleated sheet which acts as a platform and supports the two α helices. Thus, a groove or cleft is created that forms the antigen-binding site of the molecule (Figure 2.4). Most of the polymorphism of Class I molecules is found within this cleft. These differences affect the ability of a particular

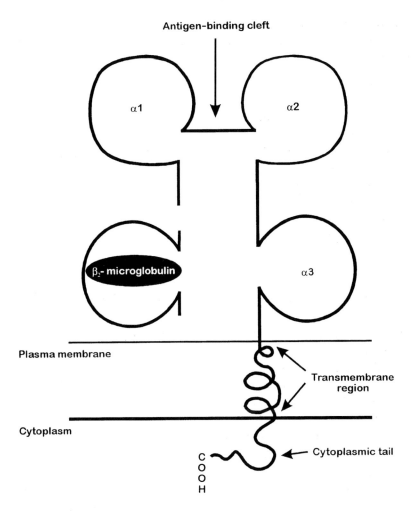

Figure 2.3 Structure of MHC Class I molecules.

Class I molecules have one glycosylated polypeptide chain encoded for by the MHC which is anchored through the cell membrane. It is non-covalently linked with another molecule — β_2-microglobulin (12 kDa) — which is not coded for by the MHC and is not membrane bound. The heavy or α chain has five distinct regions or domains, three of which are extracellular and hydrophilic (the $\alpha1$, $\alpha2$ and $\alpha3$ globular domains), one of which is transmembraneous and hydrophobic and one of which is cytoplasmic and hydrophilic

MHC Class I molecule to bind a specific processed antigen and severely restrict the range of antigens which it can present. This selectivity in antigen binding is distinct to that exhibited by immunoglobulin molecules, which exhibit exquisite specificity.

The suggestion that cytotoxic T cells (Tc) might recognise processed antigen bound to MHC Class I molecules was confirmed by a study in which target cells were pulsed with either native antigen or peptide fragments of the antigen. Only the latter sensitised the target cells to lysis by Tc. The determination of the crystal structure of HLA-A2 demonstrated a groove which could potentially bind such peptide fragments. This groove could accommodate a peptide between eight (linear) and 25 (helical) amino acids. The groove is lined by most of the polymorphic residues of the MHC Class I molecule, thus conferring the ability of different allelic forms of the molecule to bind different peptides. Analysis of the structure of naturally occurring peptides isolated from purified MHC Class I molecules demonstrated the occurrence of particular amino acid sequences that are specific to allelic forms of Class I molecules. These are likely to be important in the association between the peptide and the polymorphic residues of the Class I molecule.

The peptides which bind to the MHC Class I groove are all between 8 and 10 amino acids in length. Indeed, naturally occurring nonameric peptides bind to Class I molecules with 100–1000-fold greater affinity than peptides of any other length.

Function of Class I Molecules

As you may remember, Class I HLA molecules are present on all nucleated cells. This distribution is logical if we consider the role they play. In order for an antigen to be recognised by CD8+ T cells, it must be presented to the T cell in association with a Class I molecule. These cells play a vital role in controlling/eliminating viral infection. Since viruses may infect any cell in the body, presentation of antigen by molecules present on all body cells (except erythrocytes) means that CD8+ cells potentially can respond to all viral infections. The antigen receptor of a given T lymphocyte will recognise a particular viral peptide only in the context of a particular Class I molecule. This phenomenon is termed **HLA restriction**.

When foreign antigens are not occupying the cleft, self-antigens associate with the Class I molecules. During development in the thymus, T cells are selected according to their ability to recognise antigen in association with self-MHC molecules on the thymic epithelium. Any cells which recognise self-antigens are eliminated or inactivated, thus preventing the development of a response which would damage host tissues — **an autoimmune response**.

Class II MHC Molecules

MHC Class II molecules (HLA-DR, -DP and -DQ) are expressed on those cells capable of presenting antigen in order to stimulate an immune response. These

antigen-binding cleft

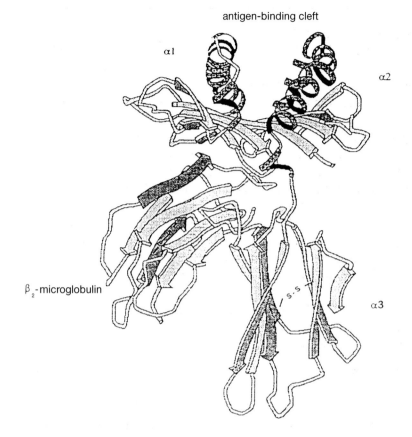

Figure 2.4 Representation of the molecular structure of an MHC Class I molecule showing the antigen-binding cleft.

Class I molecules present antigen to T cells. Each of the α1 and α2 domains consists of four β strands and an α helix. Together, these β strands form a β-pleated sheet which acts as a platform and supports the two α helices. Thus, a groove or cleft is created that forms the antigen-binding site of the molecule

include B lymphocytes, monocytes, macrophages, dendritic cells and (in humans) activated T cells. However, under appropriate conditions, cells that do not normally express Class II molecules (such as resting T cells, endothelial cells and thyroid cells) can be induced to express them.

Structure of Class II Molecules

These molecules consist of two, linked glycoproteins (α and β) composed of 229 and 237 amino acids, respectively (Figure 2.5). Both chains are coded for by the genes of the MHC. Each consists of four regions: two extracellular, hydrophilic regions (α1, α2 or β1, β2 domains), a transmembraneous, hydrophobic region

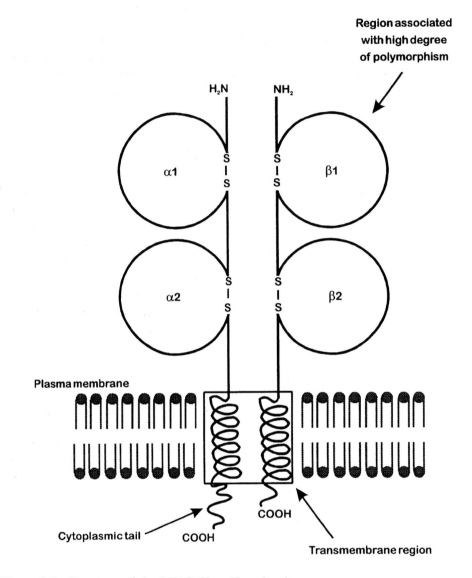

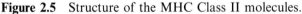

Figure 2.5   Structure of the MHC Class II molecules.

Class II molecules consist of two, linked, glycoproteins (α and β), both of which are coded for by the genes of the MHC. Each consists of four regions: two extracellular, hydrophilic regions ($\alpha 1$, $\alpha 2$ or $\beta 1$, $\beta 2$ domains), a transmembraneous, hydrophobic region and an intracellular hydrophilic region which anchors the molecule in the cell membrane

and an intracellular hydrophilic region which anchors the molecule in the cell membrane. As with MHC Class I molecules, the extracellular domains show a high degree of homology to those domains of immunoglobulin. Also, the structure created by the $\alpha 1$ and $\beta 1$ domains is composed of eight β strands and two α helices and the resulting cleft is similar to that created by the α1 and α2 domains of the Class I molecule.

The polymorphism of Class II molecules is located in the cleft, thus restricting the number of antigenic peptides which may be bound and distinguishing between the different members of this class. Like the cleft in Class I molecules, the antigen-binding site of a single Class II molecule is able to bind a range of different antigens.

Function of Class II Molecules

The receptor on CD4+ T lymphocytes recognises processed peptide associated with the cleft of a Class II molecule on an antigen-presenting cell. This recognition is constrained in a similar way to that involving CD8+ T lymphocytes and the Class I-antigen complex. However, there are differences. The peptide-binding groove of Class I molecules is closed at both ends, a feature that presumably dictates the binding of peptides of restricted size (8–10 amino acids). Class II-bound peptides are slightly larger (approximately 14 amino acids) and show heterogeneity at the carboxyl terminus, suggesting that the Class II peptide-binding groove may be open at one end.

Minor Histocompatibility Antigens

Minor histocompatibility antigens are only weakly immunogenic in a foreign host. Thus, these antigens are not usually matched in transplant patients, since the rejection reaction that they stimulate may be easily suppressed with drugs. An example of such an antigen is H-Y, which is encoded on the Y chromosome. When female mice receive grafts from males of the same strain, they may recognise the H-Y antigen and reject the graft.

THE MURINE MAJOR HISTOCOMPATIBILITY COMPLEX

The major histocompatibility complex of the mouse is formed by the H-2, Qa and TLA loci. The H-2 locus comprises a group of related genes located on chromosome 17 (Figure 2.6).

The K region of the H-2 locus encodes for a Class I antigen chain which associates with β_2-microglobulin on the surface of nearly all the cells in the mouse. The region contains more than 12 alleles. Similarly, the D region, which also encodes a Class I glycoprotein, has more than 40 alleles. The I region contains four structural genes which code for the α and β chains of the MHC Class II molecules of the mouse. The S region codes for the MHC Class III molecules. Finally, the Qa and TLA regions code for antigens which are

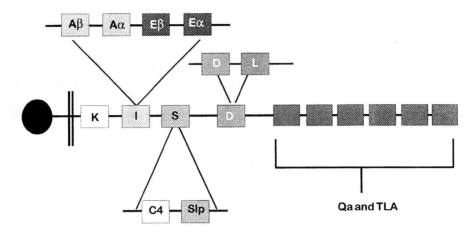

Figure 2.6   The murine major histocompatibility complex.

The major histocompatibility complex of the mouse is formed by the H-2, Qa and TLA loci. The K region of the H-2 locus encodes for a Class I antigen chain which associates with β2-microglobulin on the surface of nearly all the cells in the mouse. The D region also encodes a Class I glycoprotein. The I region genes code for the α and β chains of the MHC Class II molecules of the mouse. The S region codes for the MHC Class III molecules. Finally, the Qa and TLA regions code for antigens which are expressed on lymphocytes (Qa) and on certain leukaemia cells and immature T lymphocytes (TLA)

expressed on lymphocytes (Qa) and on certain leukaemia cells and immature T lymphocytes (TLA). These antigens are Class I molecules associated with β_2-microglobulin but their functions are unknown.

LEARNING OUTCOMES

Having completed this chapter you should have an understanding of those characteristics which make a molecule an effective immunogen. This is important from a practical point of view, since it is often necessary to raise monoclonal antibodies to different molecules in order to characterise them functionally, e.g. lymphokines. Also, such considerations are important in developing vaccines.

Additionally, you have learnt about the differences between the products of the major histocompatibility complex. The function of the MHC Class II products is discussed more fully in Chapter 5. You can test your understanding of the work covered in this chapter in the appropriate section of the accompanying program.

Chapter 3

Structures which Recognise Antigen

LEARNING OBJECTIVES

The purpose of this chapter is to introduce you to the major structures responsible for the recognition of antigens leading to an immune response and the removal of the specific antigen which originally stimulated the response. These structures include antibody, the B cell antigen receptor (BCR) and the T cell antigen receptor (TCR). We will examine their structure and function and learn the terminology associated with the molecules. It is important to remember that since antibodies are complex, proteinaceous molecules, they may also act as foreign antigens when injected into a different host. Thus, any differences between immunoglobulin molecules may be detected by examining the specificity of the antibodies raised against them. This is how the different classes and subclasses of antibodies may be distinguished.

ANTIBODIES

Antibodies are a group of glycoproteins found in the serum and body fluids. They are **gamma-globulins** and therefore are known as **immunoglobulins**.

Tiselius and Kabat (1939) showed that antibodies were gamma-globulins by incubating serum from an immune animal with specific antigen. The immune complexes formed between the antigen and antibodies precipitated out of solution and the remaining serum was analysed. The gamma-globulin portion of the serum was severely diminished.

Antibodies are also found on the surface of B cells, where they are inserted through the cell membrane (**mIg**). When B cells are activated by antigen, they proliferate and may differentiate into **plasma cells**, which manufacture large amounts of antibody. This antibody binds the same antigen as the mIg on the B cell from which the plasma cell was derived (i.e. they have the same **binding specificity**).

There are five major classes of antibody (IgG, IgA, IgM, IgE and IgD) which differ from each other in size, charge, amino acid sequence and carbohydrate content. Also, within the classes, there are distinct differences (heterogeneity), and subclasses can be distinguished, e.g. IgG_1, IgG_2, IgG_3 and IgG_4. The number of subclasses varies depending on the host species and each differs in biological function.

Antibody Structure

The basic structure of all immunoglobulins consists of two pairs of chains (heavy and light) linked together by covalent, disulphide bonds and non-covalent forces (Figure 3.1). The heavy chains dictate the class of immunoglobulin, i.e. μ chains are present in IgM, γ chains in IgG etc. The light chains may be either κ or λ type. These chains are antigenically distinct and only one type of light chain is present in any single antibody molecule. This four-chain structure is seen in IgG, IgD and IgE. By contrast, IgA occurs in both monomeric and polymeric forms (comprising more than one basic four-chain unit structure) whilst IgM occurs as a pentamer with five basic units.

Edelman received the Nobel prize for his work on determining the structure of the immunoglobulin molecule. For this purpose he used myeloma proteins. Multiple myeloma results from the uncontrolled growth of a cell which normally produces antibodies. The cell replicates unchecked and the daughter cells all produce antibody of the same type and specificity as the original cell. This leads to a high serum concentration of homologous antibody. Using this myeloma protein, Edelman identified the heavy and light chain structure of antibody molecules. After unfolding the proteins in 6 M urea, the disulphide bonds were disrupted by mercaptoethanol and prevented from re-forming by alkylation. After this treatment, he found two types of molecule with molecular masses of 20 kDa (light chain) and 50 kDa (heavy chain). Their relative concentrations suggested that the basic antibody unit consisted of two heavy chains and two light chains.

Each of the chains comprises a number of globular regions (called domains) formed by intrachain disulphide bonds. At the amino terminal of both the heavy and light chains is a single **variable region** or domain (VL or VH)

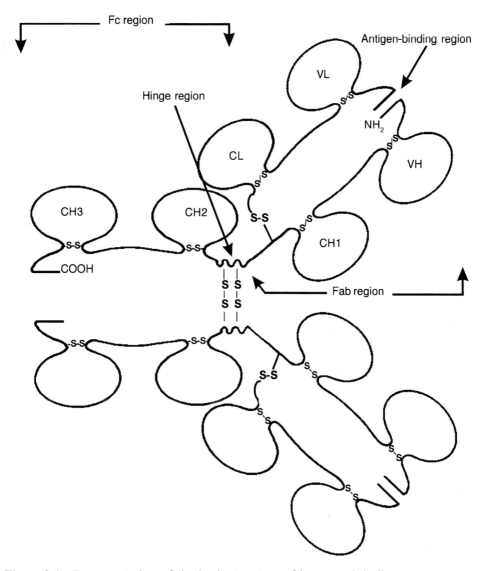

Figure 3.1   Representation of the basic structure of immunoglobulins.

   The basic structure of all immunoglobulins consists of two pairs of chains (heavy and light) linked together by covalent, disulphide bonds and non-covalent forces. Each chain comprises a number of globular regions (called domains) formed by intrachain disulphide bonds. At the amino terminal of both the heavy and light chains is a single variable region or domain (VL or VH). The number of heavy chain constant regions (CH) in an antibody molecule varies depending on the class

consisting of 110 amino acids. The variable regions of one light chain and one heavy chain form one of the antigen-binding sites of the antibody.

   The number of **heavy chain constant regions** (CH) in an antibody molecule varies, being three in IgG, IgA and IgD and four in IgM and IgE. Light chains have only one constant region (CL). These regions are called constant because there is very little difference in the secondary and tertiary structure of the proteins in these areas.

There are several genes which code for immunoglobulins and, unusually, each chain of an antibody molecule is the product of more than one of these. The variable region is coded for largely by a V gene and the constant region by a Cγ, Cμ, Cα, Cϵ or Cδ gene.

Individual CH genes are organised such that different exons code for the structural domains of the protein. Thus, the Cμ genes contain four exons to code for the four constant domains of the μ chain. The Cγ genes each have an additional small exon between the first and second CH domain exons that encodes the **hinge region**. The Cδ gene is organised somewhat differently from the other H chain genes in that it contains an extended hinge and lacks a CH2 domain.

Each class of antibody may exist in either a **secreted** or **membrane-bound** form. With the exception of IgD, the carboxy-terminal sequences of the secreted form are contiguous with the terminal C region domain. By contrast, the unique sequence of the membrane-bound form is encoded by an exon (or exons) downstream of the terminal CH exon. This sequence comprises a series of 26 hydrophobic amino acids which spans the plasma membrane, and a hydrophilic, cytoplasmic tail varying in size from 3 to 28 amino acids. For IgD, the exons for both the secreted and membrane-bound forms of the molecule are separate. The production of membrane-bound or secreted immunoglobulin is probably regulated at the level of RNA processing.

The variable regions of both the heavy and light chains are coded for by V region genes. Products of specific V region genes associate only appropriate heavy chain constant region gene products (namely the VH with CH and VL with CL gene products). However, any of the products of the CH genes may associate with any of those of the VH genes.

Kappa chains have four V region subgroups differing in the number and position of amino acid substitutions and deletions. These molecules share a degree of structural similarity which distinguishes them from lambda or VH regions. Similar subgroups also exist for lambda and heavy chain V regions.

All V gene products have regions which are relatively conserved, and it is these which define the type of the V gene product (VH or VL) and the subgroup to which it belongs. Also, they have extremely variable zones or 'hot spots'. These are the hypervariable regions which are involved in the formation of the antigen-binding site. Light chains have three hypervariable regions whilst heavy chains have four.

All antibody molecules are covalently bonded to carbohydrates in the form of simple or complex side chains. This carbohydrate may assist in secretion of the antibody by plasma cells and may affect the biological functions of the molecule which are associated with the constant regions of the heavy chains.

Antibody molecules may also be considered to consist of two functional domains: the Fab fragment (Fragment antigen binding) consists of the two VH–

CH1 domains and the two VL–CL domains; the Fc fragment (Fragment crystallisable) consists of the CH2 and CH3 domains (and CH4 in IgM and IgE) of both heavy chains. The antigen specificity of the antibody molecule resides in the Fab fragment but the majority of the biological function resides in the Fc region. These two fragments are joined by the hinge region. As its name suggests, this area allows slight relative motion between the two fragments. This mobility is important in antigen binding. The hinge region contains a high number of proline and cysteine residues; the latter form interchain disulphide bonds which maintain the integrity of the antibody molecule. These bonds also prevent folding in this area, making it especially vulnerable to enzymatic cleavage. The number of these disulphide bonds varies between classes and subclasses of antibody.

Isotypes

As we mentioned earlier, when antibodies are injected into another person or a different species, they can act as antigens, and antibodies will be raised against any part of the molecule which is foreign to the host. Thus, if human immunoglobulins are injected into mice, antibodies will form which will react with a range of epitopes on the human immunoglobulins. Isotypic antibodies react with those parts of a heavy or light chain which distinguish it from all other classes of heavy or light chains. We know that although all the immunoglobulin heavy chains have a similar structure, they have different molecular weights and therefore must have differences in their amino acid sequences and carbohydrate substitution. Thus, they must have distinguishing antigenic epitopes, which are known as **isotypes**. Antibodies may be raised to these isotypes and thus may be used to distinguish between immunoglobulin classes and subclasses.

Allotypes

In the same way that isotypic antibodies identify antigenic differences between the classes of immunoglobulins, allotypic antibodies identify antigenic determinant differences within a class (or subclass) of immunoglobulin. For example, the amino acid sequence for IgG_1 in one person (A) may vary slightly from that in another (B) due to the inheritance of different alleles of IgG_1 or to mutation. Thus, when the antibody from A is introduced into B, the differences are recognised as foreign and antibodies are formed to that part which is different — the **allotype**.

Idiotypes

In contrast to allotypic differences, idiotypic differences are associated with the antigen-binding region of an antibody. If a mouse is exposed to an antigen for the first time, it forms antibodies which have antigen-binding sites which specifically recognise the inducing antigen. If that antibody is isolated and injected into a genetically identical mouse which had not been exposed to the antigen, the only part of the antibody which would appear foreign to the recipient is the antigen-binding site. Since B cells recognise conformational antigenic determinants, the antigen-binding site (composed of the V(D)J regions of the heavy and light chains) may contain novel conformations which the recipient may recognise as foreign and to which it may form antibodies (**anti-idiotypes**). Such antibodies define the **idiotype** of the eliciting antibody. Each antigenic determinant is known as an **idiotope**.

Antibody Classes

Immunoglobulin G

IgG comprises 70–75% of the circulating immunoglobulins. It has a molecular mass of 146 kDa and a sedimentation coefficient of 7S. It is the major immunoglobulin produced during a secondary immune response and is the only antibody with antitoxin activity. It has four subclasses, IgG_1, IgG_2, IgG_3 and IgG_4. These molecules vary in molecular weight, the number and position of interchain disulphide bonds and their functional properties (Table 3.1).

IgG is the only antibody to be transported across the placenta. However, not all of the subclasses have the same properties, IgG_2 being transported more slowly than the other subclasses. One of the serum proteins which form the complement pathway—namely C1q—binds to the CH2 domain on IgG. However, the different subclasses fix C1q with reducing efficiency in the order IgG_3, IgG_1, IgG_2. Indeed, IgG_4 cannot fix C1q but may be active in the alternative complement pathway. These activities will be covered more fully in Chapter 11.

Many cells bear molecules on their surface which bind IgG through the Fc region. These are known as **Fc receptors**. The cells include phagocytes, B cells and some T cells. Fc receptors on macrophages, some T cells and killer cells allow these cells to bind antibody attached to specific antigens on cells (**target cells**) and to lyse these target cells through a mechanism known as **antibody-dependent cellular cytotoxicity (ADCC)**.

IgG is also found in mucous membrane secretions and therefore has a role to play in immunity to infection at mucosal surfaces. This activity is considered in more detail in Chapter 10.

Immunoglobulin M

IgM comprises about 10% of circulating immunoglobulins. It has a molecular mass of 970 kDa and comprises five four-chain units which are linked at the CH3 domains by inter-heavy chain disulphide bonds (Figure 3.2). The heavy

Table 3.1 General biological properties of the IgG subclasses

	IgG$_1$	IgG$_2$	IgG$_3$	IgG$_4$
% IgG in serum	60–71	19–31	5–8	0.7–4
Average serum concentration (g/l)	8	4	0.8	0.4
Range in normal serum (g/l)	5–12	2–6	0.5–1	0.2–1
% circulating B cells	40	48	8	1
Placental transfer	+ +	+	+ +	+ +
Rate of catabolism (days)	21–23	20–23	7–8	21–23
Complement fixation	+ +	+	+ +	−

chains have four constant regions and the whole unit is stabilised by a **J (joining) chain**. This immunoglobulin is largely confined to the peripheral circulation and is the principal antibody produced in a primary response. It is produced early in a secondary immune response, and in response to certain antigens is the sole antibody produced, e.g. natural blood group antibodies. IgM, with IgD, is found on the surface of the majority of B cells. It is the most efficient antibody at complement fixation; one molecule bound to antigen will initiate the complement cascade.

Immunoglobulin A

IgA comprises about 15–20% of the circulating immunoglobulin pool. In humans, the majority of serum IgA (80%) occurs as a basic four-chain monomeric unit. However, in other mammals it occurs chiefly as a dimer which is held together by a J chain synthesised by plasma cells.

IgA is the chief antibody secreted at mucous membranes, where it exists predominantly as a dimer of molecular mass 385 kDa (Figure 3.3). Dimeric IgA with its associated J chain passes through the epithelial cell layers, where it acquires the **secretory component**. This is bound by strong covalent bonds, aids release of the dimer at mucosal surfaces and protects it from proteolytic attack. Mucosal IgA probably exerts its protective effect by blocking access of the antigen to the immune system rather than by destroying it.

There are at least two different subclasses of IgA, both of which, like IgM, have an extra heavy chain constant region. Neither of the subclasses activates complement via the classical pathway, but both may activate the alternative pathway. IgA$_1$ predominates in serum but IgA$_2$ predominates in mucous secretions. This may be related to the fact that many micro-organisms release proteases capable of cleaving IgA$_1$ (e.g. meningococci).

Immunoglobulin D

Although IgD comprises less than 1% of serum immunoglobulin, it is expressed (with IgM) in the surface membrane of many B cells. This expression appears to

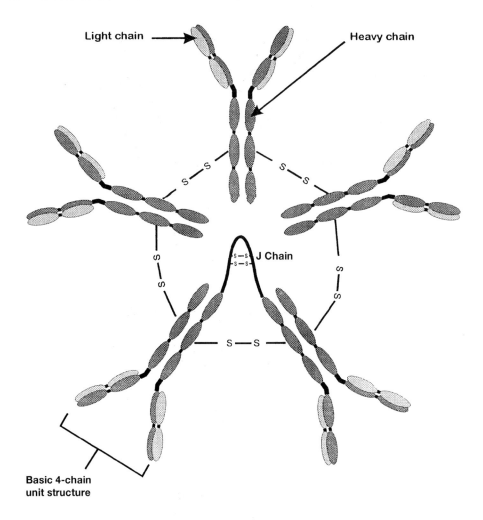

Figure 3.2   Representation of the structure of immunoglobulin M.
    IgM comprises five four-chain units which are linked at the CH3 domains by inter-heavy chain disulphide bonds. The heavy chains have four constant regions and the whole unit is stabilised by a J (joining) chain

indicate the differentiation of a pre-B cell into a mature B cell. The biological role of IgD is largely unknown but the molecule is thought to be involved in antigen-triggered lymphocyte differentiation. IgD has a tendency to undergo spontaneous proteolysis and is more sensitive to proteolytic cleavage than IgG_1, IgG_2, IgA or IgM. It is also easily destroyed by heat.

Immunoglobulin E

Only trace amounts of IgE are present in the serum; the majority of this antibody is bound to the surface of mast cells and basophils. It is functionally

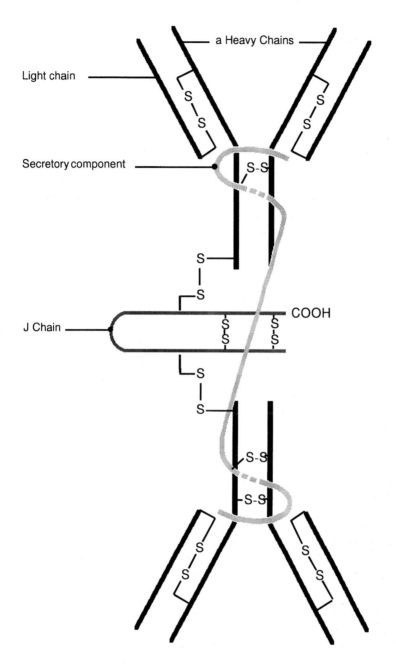

Figure 3.3   Representation of the structure of secretory immunoglobulin A.
    In humans, the majority of IgA occurs as a basic four-chain monomeric unit.
However, when it is secreted at mucous membranes, it exists predominantly as a dimer
which is held together by a J chain. On passing through the epithelial cell layers it
acquires the secretory component. This is bound by strong covalent bonds and aids
release of the dimer at mucosal surfaces

associated with those reactions that occur in individuals who are undergoing an allergic reaction. It can activate the alternative complement pathway. IgE also has a role to play in immunity to helminthic infections. Along with IgM, IgE has an extra heavy chain constant domain.

Antibody Function

Functionally, antibodies show a spectrum of activities, ranging from those which are beneficial (such as the neutralisation of viruses) to those which cause damage to the host (such as the prevention of nervous impulse conduction in myasthenia gravis). These functions are covered in more detail in the appropriate chapters and a summary is given in Table 3.2.

Fc receptors

As mentioned earlier, certain cells express surface membrane receptors which bind the Fc region of immunoglobulins. These Fc receptors (FcR) may be classified according to the class of antibody they bind, e.g. $Fc\varepsilon R$ (IgE receptor) and $Fc\alpha R$ (IgA receptor) and $Fc\gamma R$ (IgG receptor). The $Fc\gamma R$ may be divided further into three groups—$Fc\gamma RI$, $Fc\gamma RII$, $Fc\gamma RIII$—which differ in their

Table 3.2 Summary of the biological functions of immunoglobulin

Function	Description
Neutralisation	Antibodies may block cellular receptors for toxins, bacteria or viruses, preventing toxicity/infection
Complement fixation	Activation of the classical pathway occurs as a result of complement components binding to the CH2 region of Ig
Opsonisation	Phagocytosis of an object is greatly enhanced when it is coated by antibodies—a process known as opsonisation
Allergy and anaphylaxis	Antigen-specific IgE may bind to receptors on mast cells and promote their degranulation, leading to the signs and symptoms of allergy
Antibody-dependent cellular cytotoxicity	Antibodies stimulated by virus infection bind to viral antigens expressed on the surface of infected cells. The Fc portion binds to FcR-bearing cells which are able to lyse the virally infected cells
Agglutination	Each antibody molecule has at least two sites to which antigen can bind. Thus they may 'stick together' or agglutinate a number of organisms
Effect on microbial physiology	Some antibodies inhibit the movement of organisms by attaching to flagella. Also, some antibodies inhibit the metabolism or growth of micro-organisms

affinity for IgG and immune complexes. The properties and cellular distribution of these receptors are summarised in Table 3.3.

THE B CELL ANTIGEN RECEPTOR

As mentioned before, B cells bind antigen via membrane-bound immunoglobulin molecules (mIg). Normal B cells in the peripheral blood have 10^4–10^5 antibody molecules in their membrane which differ from the secreted form due to the presence of spacer, transmembrane and cytoplasmic sequences at the Fc (carboxyl) end of the heavy chains. When antigen binds to mIg, the cell must be made aware of this event. This is achieved through a series of biochemical events collectively known as **signal transduction**. This is usually achieved by the interaction of particular cellular proteins (e.g. G proteins or tyrosine kinase) with specific regions of the cytoplasmic tails of mIg. However, the most prevalent mIgs, IgM and IgD, do not possess such regions in their tails, suggesting that the required signals are transmitted in some other way. Other similar receptor systems have been shown to have associated proteins which

Table 3.3 Summary of the function and distribution of Fc receptors for IgG

Receptor	Molecular mass	Function	Cellular distribution
FcγRI (CD 64)	72 kDa	Binds monomeric IgG; high-affinity receptor; binds IgG in CH2 region; important in clearance of immune complexes and ADCC	Monocytes, macrophages. Expression is increased on monocytes treated with the cytokine interferon-gamma
FcγRII (CDw32)	40 kDa	Low-affinity receptor for aggregated IgG; occupation triggers IgG-mediated phagocytosis and triggers an oxidative burst in monocytes and neutrophils; simultaneous binding to mIg and occupation of FcγRII on B cells provides a negative signal	FcγRII comprises a group of proteins coded by a number of closely related genes. All types are expressed on monocytes, FcγRIIB is present on B cells and FcγRIIB and C are expressed by neutrophils
FcγRIII (CD 16)	50–80 kDa	Low-affinity receptor for aggregated IgG; mediates phagocytosis and ADCC	There are two distinct forms of FcγRIII, a transmembrane form and a glycosyl-phosphatidyl-inositol-linked form (GPI-linked form). The transmembrane form is expressed on macrophages and NK cells, the GPI-linked form on neutrophils

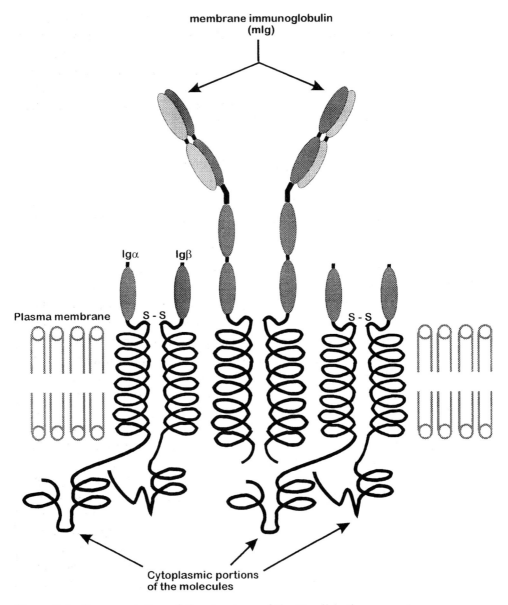

Figure 3.4   Representation of the structure of the T cell antigen receptor.

mIg on the surface of B cells is non-covalently associated with a dimeric protein consisting of two disulphide-linked glycoproteins. These molecules are known as Igα and Igβ

perform the task of signal transduction, and recent studies have demonstrated the presence of novel mIg-associated transmembrane proteins on B cells. mIgM is non-covalently associated with a dimeric protein consisting of two disulphide-linked glycoproteins. These molecules have become known as Igα and Igβ and have molecular masses of about 32–33 kDa and 37 kDa (Figure 3.4). In the mouse, a further chain exists, the Igγ with a molecular mass of 34 kDa. The amino acid sequences of the chains indicate that both Igα and Igβ have a single, extracellular domain which shows similarity in both sequence and structure to those in immunoglobulin molecules. Thus, the genes coding for all these molecules (**mb-1** for Igα and **B29** for Igβ and Igγ) are considered to belong to the same family, which has become known as the **immunoglobulin supergene family**. We will come across more members of this family shortly.

THE T CELL RECEPTOR

The identity of the molecule on the surface of T cells which binds antigen took many years to determine. T cells had been shown experimentally to exhibit

The development of antigen-specific T cell clones (T cells derived from a single antigen-reactive cell which therefore recognise the same antigenic determinant) allowed the structure of the T cell antigen receptor to be determined. Basically, cloned, antigen-specific T cells were injected into a mouse and monoclonal antibodies were produced. Antibodies which recognised determinants expressed only by the cells used to immunise the mice were identified. Since the only difference between these and other T cells should be the molecules which recognise antigen, the monoclonal antibodies were assumed to recognise the T cell antigen receptor (TCR). Partial confirmation of this was obtained by incubating the T cell clone with the monoclonal antibody and then stimulating with antigen. The antibody blocked antigen recognition and the cells failed to proliferate. The antibody was used to isolate the receptor by labelling cells, lysing them and incubating them with the monoclonal antibody. The immune complexes were then removed by reacting them with a substance that binds the Fc region of Ig (protein A) and analysed by sodium dodecyl sulphate polyacrylamide gel electrophoresis (SDS-PAGE). The proteins from the cells were labelled with a radioactive substance. Thus, when the SDS-PAGE gels were exposed to film, bands containing cell-derived proteins could be visualised.

antigen specificity and so it seemed logical that they must express antigen-specific receptors. Finally, the T cell antigen receptor (TCR) was identified by using antibodies with unique specificity for a particular clone of T cells as an 80–90-kDa, cell surface, dimeric glycoprotein (Figure 3.5). The disulphide-linked α and β chains each consisted of two extracellular domains, one constant and one variable, with a joining segment in between. A short cytoplasmic tail connects the extracellular domains via a transmembraneous region, which is

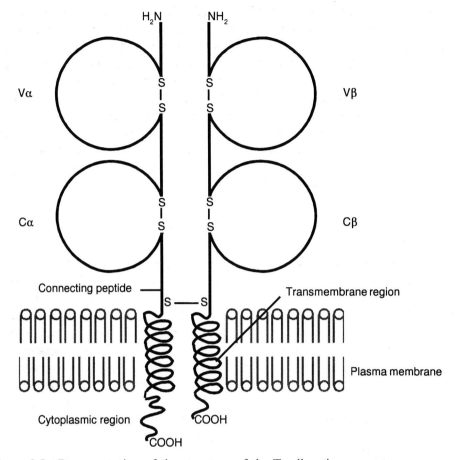

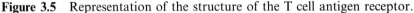

Figure 3.5 Representation of the structure of the T cell antigen receptor.
The TCR is a cell surface, dimeric glycoprotein. The disulphide-linked α and β chains each consist of two extracellular domains, one constant and one variable, with a joining segment in between. A short cytoplasmic tail connects the extracellular domains via a transmembraneous region. The variable regions of the α and β chains together form the antigen-binding site of the receptor

next to a group of about 20 amino acids (containing cysteines) which comprise the connecting peptide where the interchain disulphide bridges are probably formed.

The variable regions of the α and β chains together form the antigen-binding site of the receptor. Amino acid sequence analysis suggests that the variable regions show a β-pleated sheet structure similar to that seen in the variable regions of antibody molecules. Within the variable domain, at least three hypervariable regions have been identified which are directly involved in antigen binding. The structural similarity between antibody molecules and the TCR chains have led to the inclusion of the genes coding for the TCR in the Ig supergene family.

Following the identification of the $\alpha\beta$TCR, cells were isolated which expressed a different chain — the γ chain (55 kDa). Although similar to the $\alpha\beta$ molecules, the γ chain lacks glycosylation. It was found to be non-covalently associated with a protein of molecular mass 40 kDa — the δ chain. The $\gamma\delta$TCR is expressed on a proportion of mature T cells and thymocytes; its presence precludes the expression of the $\alpha\beta$TCR. Although their distribution is similar, in humans, cells expressing the $\gamma\delta$TCR are far less common than those expressing the $\alpha\beta$TCR. The major function ascribed to the $\gamma\delta$TCR+ cells is **MHC-unrestricted cellular cytotoxicity**. In this respect, $\gamma\delta$TCR+ cells are more like NK cells than cytotoxic T cells. The $\gamma\delta$ receptor may recognise antigens associated with non-classical MHC molecules.

The CD3 Complex

As mentioned earlier, the TCR was identified by precipitation of labelled cell membrane-associated proteins using monoclonal antibodies. When different detergents were used and the precipitated proteins separated by two-dimensional electrophoresis, sequentially under non-reducing and reducing conditions, further molecules (γ, δ, ε, ζ) were identified which associated with the TCR (Figure 3.6). Originally these were known as the **T3 complex** and subsequently as the **CD3 complex**. Later work identified a further two molecules associated with CD3, the ω chain (which may be detected in the cytoplasm of T cells) and the Υ chain. More recently, it has been concluded that the ζ and η chains do not form part of the CD3 complex but are involved in relaying information from the TCR–CD3 complex to the cell.

CD3 molecules are expressed on a proportion of thymocytes and on all peripheral T cells in association with the TCR chains. Their presence is vital for the expression of the TCR chains and thus for the presence of a functional receptor on the cell membrane.

Ohashi et al (1985) showed that mutant cells which have lost the ability to express one or other of the TCR genes have neither the TCRα chain nor the CD3 complex on their membranes. If the cells are transfected with a competent β chain gene, the cells are able to express a functional $\alpha\beta$TCR and the CD3 complex.

Experiments have shown that it is not only the physical expression of CD3 and TCR that are linked; they appear to be functionally linked also. Experiments have shown that antibodies that bind CD3 (anti-CD3 antibodies) may inhibit the proliferation of antigen-specific T cells, probably by causing **capping** (movement of a molecule within the plane of the membrane to the pole of the

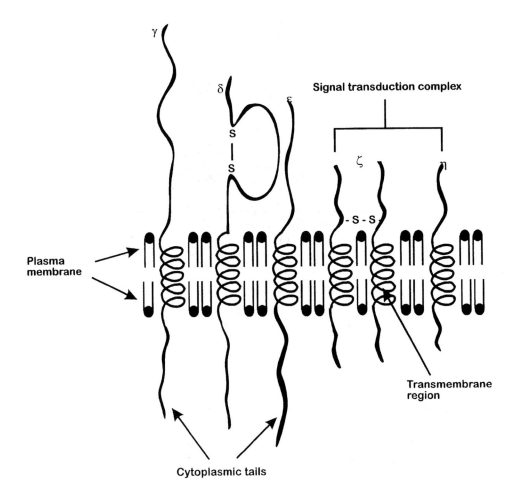

Figure 3.6   The molecular make-up of the CD3 complex.
  CD3 molecules are expressed on a proportion of thymocytes and on all peripheral T cells in association with the TCR chains. Their presence is vital for the expression of the TCR chains and thus for the presence of a functional receptor on the cell membrane

cell) and **recycling** of CD3. It has been shown that the TCR co-caps with CD3. Thus, this treatment would reduce expression of the antigen receptor and thereby inhibit antigen-induced activation. Conversely, anti-CD3 has been shown to stimulate cells when it is anchored to a solid support. It is thought that, in this form, the antibody is able to cross-link TCR–CD3 complexes and thus provide a similar signal to that which is delivered when antigen binds the TCR.
  The γ, δ and ε chains of CD3 are non-covalently linked, transmembraneous polypeptides. The molecules of CD3 are thought to associate with the $\alpha\beta$ chains of the TCR so that an ε molecule associates with each chain of the TCR (Figure 3.7). The transmembrane regions of both the δ and ε chains of CD3 have

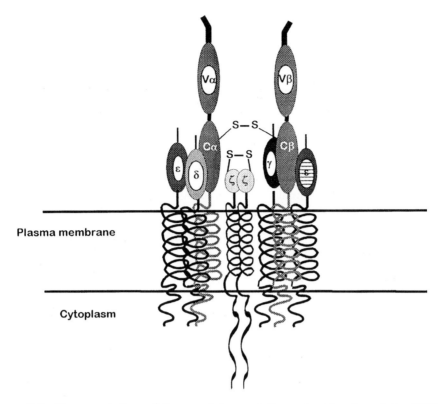

Figure 3.7 Representation of the spacial association of molecules of the TCR and CD3 complex.

The γ, δ and ε chains of CD3 are non-covalently linked, transmembraneous polypeptides and are thought to associate with the $\alpha\beta$ chains of the TCR so that an ε molecule associates with each chain of the TCR

aspartate molecules which may form salt bridges with lysine molecules in the equivalent part of the TCR chains.

Function of the TCR–CD3 Complex

As its title suggests, the TCR is responsible for recognising a specific antigen and the CD3 complex provides the appropriate information to the cell concerning this interaction.

In order for a cell to respond to a specific antigen, the 'nerve centre' of the cell must 'know' when an antigen has interacted with its receptor. This information is relayed (signal transduction) by a series of chemical messengers from the membrane to the appropriate places within the cell such that a suitable response may be given (e.g. production of lymphokines). Since only a short portion of the composite chains of the TCR extends into the cytoplasm of the cell, it is thought that CD3 and/or the $\zeta\eta$ molecules are responsible for signal transduction.

LEARNING OUTCOMES

Having studied this chapter you should have a good understanding of the structure and function of those molecules responsible for recognising antigen on lymphocytes. You should understand the differences between the various classes of antibody and how secreted antibody differs from that found on the surface of B cells. An important aspect of this chapter is the introduction of the immunoglobulin supergene family. Many biologically important molecules belong to this family and have structural similarities, which means that they often show similar functional characteristics or have similar signal transduction pathways associated with them. You should now test yourself to see if you have understood the information provided in this chapter.

Chapter 4

The Generation of Antibody and T Cell Antigen Receptor Diversity

LEARNING OBJECTIVES

The immune system is exposed to an enormous variety of antigens in the form of infectious agents and must be able to respond to such a challenge. However, the number of genes required to code for every possible antigenic determinant would be enormous. Thus, logically, a balance is required. Since it is important that the immune system does not react to self-antigens, the range of possible antibody specificities (the antibody repertoire) must be great enough to prevent extensive cross-reactivity between self-antigens and those on infectious agents but small enough that there is space for the genetic material required. This logic must also be extended to the T cell antigen receptor, where the specificity is not as exquisite as that found in antibodies but must be great enough to allow some distinction between antigens. In this chapter we shall discover how this balance has been achieved and how the specificity of an immune response is controlled.

THEORIES CONCERNING ANTIBODY DIVERSITY

Although there is some heterogeneity in the constant region of immunoglobulin heavy chains (which has given rise to the classes and subclasses of immunoglobulins), the major cause for heterogeneity in the total immuno-globulin population is due to that of the variable regions. The number of genes determining this diversity remains controversial.

Over the years, many theories have been proposed to explain the range of antigenic determinants recognised by antibodies. Two particular theories received the most attention and have been given greatest credence. The **germ line theory** proposes that there must be a gene in the germ line (i.e. the original chromosome complement present at conception) to code for every antibody variable region and that these genes arose by **duplication** during evolution. By contrast, the **somatic mutation theory** proposes that only a small number of variable region genes are present in the germ line and that the products of these genes may vary greatly due to **point mutation** or **recombination** during lymphocyte differentiation, thus giving rise to a unique antibody repertoire in each person. If diversity were dependent on this theory alone, there would have to exist special mechanisms for selecting variants, due to the normally low rate of mutation. Recent studies using DNA cloning techniques suggest that both of the theories contribute to antibody diversity but the relative contribution of each in generating antibody diversity remains unknown.

THE GENETIC BASIS OF ANTIBODY DIVERSITY

During B cell development, rearrangement of Ig genes results in the surface membrane expression of antibody with a single antigenic specificity. Although there may be more than one type of antibody expressed on the surface of a single B cell (commonly IgM and IgD are co-expressed), all the molecules use the same VH and VL genes. The antigen-binding site of an antibody is made up of the **V(ariability)**, **D(iversity)** and **J(oining)** regions of the **heavy chain** and the **VJ** regions of the **light chain** (Figure 4.1). Immunoglobulin diversity is affected by a variety of genetic mechanisms but the number of VH, VL, DH, JH and JL genes is highly influential.

V, D and J Region Heavy Chain Genes

DNA sequence and Southern blotting analyses have resulted in the VH region being divided into seven or eight subfamilies, each having between four and more than 100 members. However, recent work has suggested that this severely underestimates the number of VH genes present in the germ line.

Currently, in humans, there are thought to be between 10 and 20 D region genes and nine J region genes (including three pseudogenes). Mice apparently only have four genes in this region.

Light Chain V and J Genes

Unlike their counterparts in heavy chains, light chains do not contain D regions. The V region is divided into a leader exon and one further exon which codes for the bulk of the V region. In mice, the V region comprises two alleles, each of which is associated with two J region alleles. In contrast to this, the number of genes in the human Vλ region is much greater than in mice, which may reflect the greater usage of the L chain in humans.

The Vκ locus in both humans and mice comprises a number of Vκ genes (estimated to be between 50 and 300 in humans) and five Jκ genes. Analysis using Southern blotting has allowed the subdivision of Vκ genes into families similar to those of the VH genes.

GENERATION OF ANTIBODY DIVERSITY

The **primary antibody repertoire** of an individual includes the specificity of all those antibodies which normally circulate in the bloodstream. They do not result from exposure to specific antigen and arise through the random combination of immunoglobulin heavy and light chain V, D and J segments; a process resulting in **combinatorial diversity**. However, the repertoire is

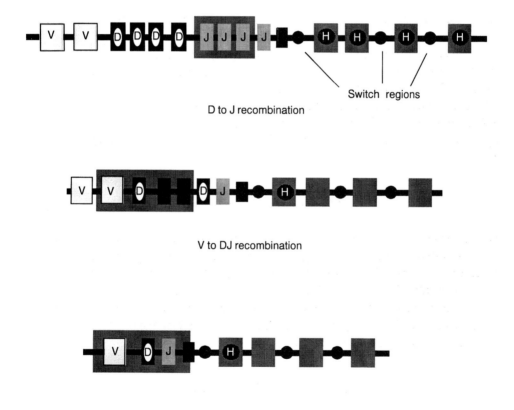

Figure 4.1 Genetic make-up of the antigen-binding site of antibody molecules.

The antigen-binding site of an antibody is made up of the V(ariability), D(iversity) and J(oining) regions of the heavy chain and the VJ regions of the light chain. The number of VH, VL, DH, JH and JL genes influences the diversity of the antibody response due to recombination between the different genes

increased further as a result of the imprecision in joining the different gene segments, i.e. **junctional diversity**. Since each amino acid is coded for by a group of three bases, errors in joining gene segments together may result in a **frame shift** or the replacement of one amino acid by another. This may lead to a conformational change which will affect the binding specificity of the antibody.

Studies in mice have shown that the bone marrow produces enough primary B cells every few days to completely renew the peripheral blood pool. These cells, if they do not encounter antigen, have a short life of between 4 and 7 days. Thus, the B cell antigen-recognition repertoire is constantly changing through the production of cells which are using different VDJ gene combinations. Thus, in an infection, if none of the primary B cells expresses an antibody which recognises the antigen, it is likely that one with effective affinity will be produced within a few days through combinatorial and junctional diversity.

Following exposure to an antigen, reactive B cells undergo a process of **hypermutation** within the Ig gene loci. This results in the maturation of the immune response, with the production of antibodies of increased affinity. However, only a minor proportion of the point mutations which occur actually contribute to the observed increase in antibody affinity. These processes will be discussed more fully below.

Combinatorial and Junctional Diversity

Before the genetic code for an antibody is transcribed, segments of the Ig gene loci are rearranged in a two-step process to give rise to the code for the functional protein. First, a particular D region gene associates with a J region gene. The second step results in a V region gene being associated with the rearranged DJ genes. The multiplicity of genes in each region gives rise to a wide range of different combinations (Table 4.1), i.e. combinatorial diversity. In pre-B cells, those VH genes closest to the JH genes are preferentially recombined. However, this preference does not persist in mature B cells, suggesting that **antigenic pressure** may affect the VH repertoire.

Table 4.1   Estimate of the number of different antibody specificities possible through combinatorial diversity

	IgH	Igκ
V region genes	1000	200
D region genes	15	—
J region genes	4	4
Combinatorial joining	6×10^4	8×10^2
Combinatorial association	$\sim 5 \times 10^7$	

Further diversity is introduced into the antibody repertoire through the imprecision of the joining process. The point at which V, D and J gene segments join may differ by as much as 10 bases, which may result in removal of nucleotides from the ends of the regions, leading to codon changes and amino acid differences in the processed protein (junctional diversity). The result of this imprecision is that the majority of the gene rearrangements are non-productive, because the joining has resulted in non-translatable base sequences. However, if the joining process is productive (i.e. the joins are 'in frame'), each cell undergoes further gene rearrangement involving the L chain, V and J region genes. Once the L chain genes have been productively rearranged and a functional antibody has been assembled, further H and L chain rearrangement is prevented, thus ensuring that the cell produces mIg of a single specificity.

Since the antigen-binding region of an antibody is formed by both the VH and VL regions, further diversity can be introduced through the association of different rearranged heavy and light chain regions, i.e. combinatorial association. However, some VH and VL combinations prevent the association of functional H and L chains. Such failure to produce functional antibodies could be very wasteful and thus, during maturation, L chain gene rearrangement only ceases once a fully assembled, functional protein is produced.

Further diversity may be introduced in the variable regions of heavy (but not light) chains through the addition of nucleotides which are not coded for by either of the gene segments to be joined. The insertion of these **N regions** correlates with the level of activity of an enzyme called **terminal deoxynucleotidyl transferase (TdT)**, and their compositions reflect the preference of this enzyme for guanosine nucleotides.

Control of VDJ Gene Rearrangement

It has been shown that the V, D and J gene segments are flanked by either a conserved series of seven bases or a less conserved nine-base sequence. These regions are separated by a spacer whose length is either 12 or 23 bases (which approximates to one or two turns of the double helix). It is the length, rather than the sequence, of the spacer which directs recombination, since a segment with a 12-base spacer can only recombine with a segment containing a 23-base spacer (the '12–23' rule). This means that VH–D and D–JH joins may occur, whilst VH–JH association may not. However, rearrangement of VH region genes to non-rearranged D region genes is not normally seen, suggesting that there must be other mechanisms controlling the VDJ rearrangement.

Two recombination-activating genes have been identified (**RAG-1** and **RAG-2**), and whilst there is no direct, convincing evidence that the products of these genes participate in the events leading to recombination, strong, indirect evidence suggests that they form an essential part of the **recombinase enzyme** complex (e.g. no V(D)J recombination has been demonstrated in the absence of RAG-1 or RAG-2).

Mechanisms of V(D)J Rearrangement

As we mentioned earlier, the gene sequences to be joined are flanked on either side by either a heptamer or nonamer and are separated by a spacer region. These flanking sequences with the intervening spacer are together known as the **recombination signal sequence (RSS)**, which is removed in the joining process. Commonly, gene segments are joined by a **deletional method**, where the intervening DNA is **looped out** and lost from the genome (Figure 4.2a). However, not all recombination can be accounted for in this way, and some may result from **inversion** or **unequal sister chromatid exchange** (Figure 4.2b,c).

Diversity Due to Somatic Mutation

During the later stages of B cell maturation, antibody diversity is increased further through **somatic mutation**. This results in single-base changes throughout the VH and VL regions. However, certain areas within these regions are particularly susceptible to somatic mutation. Such mutation is thought to increase the affinity of the antibody for its antigen and thus to contribute to maturation of the antibody response. For example, it is probable that those B cells which proliferate, particularly in limiting antigen concentration, have undergone somatic mutation and as a result have membrane immunoglobulin with higher affinity for antigen.

Antibody Maturation

Antibody maturation is restricted to T-dependent antigens and is brought about in one of two ways: (i) the germ line genes used in the primary response are different to those used in a memory response; (ii) diversification of the primary repertoire is enhanced through repeated mutation leading to random changes in both heavy and light chain genes which occasionally result in increased affinity of the antibody for its antigen. Cells producing these higher-affinity antibodies preferentially differentiate into memory cells.

THE T CELL ANTIGEN RECEPTOR

T cell antigen receptor (TCR) diversity is generated in a manner similar to that observed with membrane immunoglobulin. A large number of genes have been identified in the germ line which contribute to TCR diversity in conjunction with that produced as a result of recombination. However, in contrast to the generation of antibody diversity, TCR diversity is rarely, if ever, affected by somatic mutation.

a) Deletion

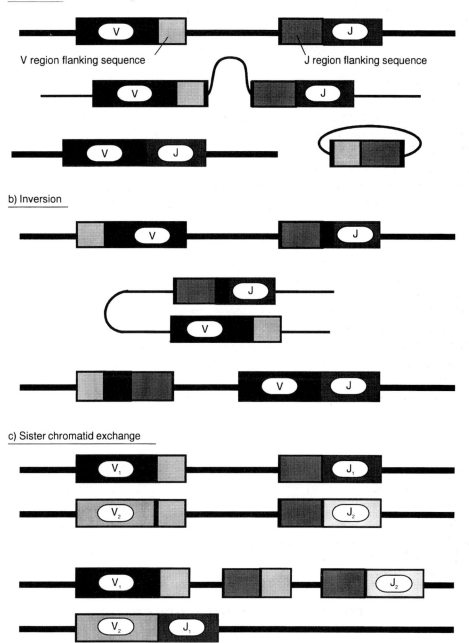

V region flanking sequence

J region flanking sequence

b) Inversion

c) Sister chromatid exchange

Figure 4.2   Methods of gene recombination which give diversity to the antibody response.

Commonly, gene segments are joined by a deletional method where the intervening DNA is looped out and lost from the genome (a). However, not all recombination can be accounted for in this way and some may result from inversion (b) or unequal sister chromatid exchange (c)

Like antibodies, the TCR is coded for by variability (V) and joining (J) region genes but lacks diversity (D) region genes in all but one of the identified components (the β chain). Whilst the TCR repertoire used in response to a particular antigen may be quite diverse, studies have shown that such responses may also be extremely restricted. Such restriction reflects not only limited V and J gene usage (for both α and β chains) but also relatively conserved amino acid usage in the junctional regions. In contrast to this, it has been shown that diverse responses reflect unrestricted usage of V and J region genes (apart from the preferential use of certain Vβ genes), and heterogeneous amino acid composition in the junctional regions of both α and β chains. These extremes may be explained by the 'similarity to self' rule.

'Similarity to Self' Rule

Limited TCR Repertoire

When an antigen is similar to one or more normally present in the body, the T cell repertoire is limited. This is to reduce the possibility of the foreign antigen stimulating cross-reactive T cells which recognise self-proteins and thus minimise the risk of developing an autoimmune response (i.e. one which recognises and destroys antigens present in the normal healthy body, thus leading to tissue damage, disease and possibly death).

Diverse TCR Repertoire

An infectious agent may have a wide range of antigenic determinants. The development of a diverse TCR repertoire in response to microbial infection is advantageous to the host, since this would increase the rate of patient survival and decrease the likelihood of the pathogens escaping recognition. Rapidly replicating micro-organisms undergo mutations relatively frequently, and if such a mutation were to affect the only antigenic determinant recognised by a limited TCR repertoire, the micro-organism would be able to grow unchecked. However, if the TCR repertoire were diverse enough to recognise several determinants on a single organism, such mutation would not prevent elimination of the infection (Figure 4.3).

GENOMIC ORGANISATION OF THE TCR

The TCRα Chain

The TCRα gene locus comprises a single constant region gene associated with a group of Jα and Vα genes. The extracellular part of the constant region, which

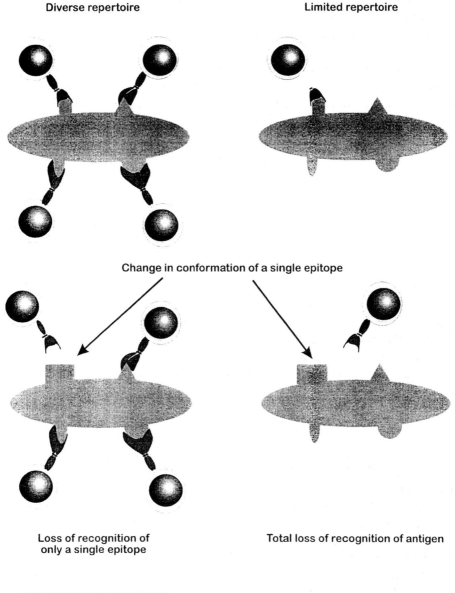

Diverse repertoire   **Limited repertoire**

Change in conformation of a single epitope

Loss of recognition of
only a single epitope

Total loss of recognition of antigen

ELIMINATION OF INFECTION

PERSISTENCE OF INFECTION

Figure 4.3   Dependence on TCR diversity for the elimination of infection.
Micro-organisms are constantly undergoing mutation. If the TCR showed a limited repertoire, mutation in a dominant antigen on the micro-organism would prevent its recognition by T cells and lead to persistent infection. Such a mutation will not prevent elimination if the T cell repertoire is diverse enough to recognise alternative epitopes on the micro-organism

includes a short connecting peptide, is coded for by two exons; a third exon codes for the transmembrane region and intracellular cytoplasmic tail. The numerous Jα region genes (estimated to be about 50) are spread out along the genome, the entire locus extending over about 100 000 bases. Despite difficulties in estimating the size of the Vα germ line repertoire, in both mouse and human it has been calculated to comprise 50–100 gene segments, divided into at least 10 different subfamilies which range in size from 1 to 10 members.

The TCRβ Chain

The genome which codes for the TCRβ chain contains a duplicated set of one Cβ and D region gene and several J region genes. The two Cβ genes are highly conserved, with only four amino acid differences in the mouse and six in humans. They have identical organisation, being encoded by four exons. The first exon encodes the extracellular constant region domain and part of the connecting peptide, the remainder of which is encoded by the second exon and part of the third exon. The transmembrane region is encoded by the remainder of the third exon and the cytoplasmic tail by the fourth exon.

Each D region gene (Dβ1 and Dβ2) is located about 600 bases from its J region gene segment (Jβ1 and Jβ2 comprising six and seven genes respectively). The Vβ region comprises about 20 genes in the mouse and 50–100 genes in the human. Part of the translated V region (about 15–17 amino acids) is coded for by genes of the J region.

The TCRγ Chain

The organisation of the genome for the TCRγ chain is complex. Humans have two Cγ genes about 16 000 bases apart. Each of these genes consists of three exons; one codes for the extracellular domain and the second codes for the majority of the connecting peptide. The third exon also encodes the extracellular domain as well as the remainder of the connecting peptide, the transmembrane region and the cytoplasmic tail. In mice there are four Cγ genes.

In humans, three Jγ gene segments have been identified associated with one of the Cγ gene segments, and two with the other. All of these genes have been shown to be used by T cell clones. By contrast, in mice, each C gene is associated with a single J gene. No Dγ gene segments have been demonstrated in either the human or murine genomes.

Eight Vγ genes have been identified in humans. These are located upstream of the two Cγ genes. In mice, there are seven Vγ genes associated, one with each of the first three Cγ genes and four with the last.

The TCRδ Chain

The δ chain is coded for by a constant gene segment and at least one J and one D gene segment. These genes are located between the variable and joining region genes of the α chain and have been shown to use some of the latter during recombination.

GENERATION OF TCR DIVERSITY

As stated earlier, the mechanisms involved in the generation of diversity in the T cell antigen receptor are similar to those found in B cells, i.e. gene duplication in the germ line coupled with combinatorial diversity and joining diversity. As with antibodies, gene rearrangement during TCR transcription is controlled by the '12–23 rule', which allows Vβ–Dβ–Jβ, Vβ–Jβ and even Dβ–Dβ joining.

   As with antibodies, TCR gene rearrangement results in substantial junctional diversity due to the lack of precision in the joining process. This is particularly important for generating diversity in the TCRγ chains, which have a comparatively small number of genes in the germ line. Also, N region diversity of the variable regions has been shown in α, β and γ chains of the TCR. As with antibodies, terminal deoxynucleotidyl transferase (TdT) has been associated with this process in T cells and is found to be highly active in the thymus, where the TCR repertoire is generated.

THE SIZE OF THE T CELL REPERTOIRE

As with antibodies, the size of the TCR repertoire may be estimated by considering the number of V(D) and J region genes and their possible combinations. However, due to the elimination of autoreactive T cells in the thymus and the requirement for MHC restriction, the repertoire expressed in the periphery is less than that estimated using these values.

LEARNING OUTCOMES

This chapter has introduced you to the terminology and the mechanisms involved in how the immune system generates a diverse enough repertoire to cope with any foreign invader it might encounter. It also introduces you to the concept of antibody affinity and maturation. These are important phenomena in the containment and elimination of infection. Thus, it is important that you understand exactly how the recombination events occur and are controlled and how this leads to a highly specific immune response. These subjects are covered in great detail in the Further Reading.

Chapter 5

Complement
and the
Inflammatory Response

LEARNING OBJECTIVES

The term **inflammation** encompasses a complex series of cellular and chemical interactions which limit the spread of an infection and the resultant tissue damage. However, the very nature of the reaction to infection or tissue damage means that the inflammatory response itself may result in tissue damage (a reaction often referred to as **hypersensitivity**). Owing to the highly reactive agents released by cells during an inflammatory response the outcome may be dramatic at best and, at worst, life-threatening. Some of these agents — **anaphylatoxins** — which are involved in an extreme response known as **anaphylactic shock** are derived from certain serum proteins which form part of the **complement cascade**.

This chapter is designed to introduce you to the concept of inflammation and its regulation and the component parts of this complex reaction, including the complement cascade. We shall discuss the activation and regulation of this group of proteins and the role each plays in non-specific immunity.

THE COMPLEMENT CASCADE

Complement is a term used to describe a group of serum and cell surface proteins which have a number of important functions, including lysis of cells and micro-organisms, opsonisation of micro-organisms (a mechanism which increases phagocytosis), and regulation of inflammatory and immune responses. Owing to these wide-ranging and often dramatic effects, the complement components are present as inactive precursors in the blood.

There are two major pathways by which complement may be activated. These are the **classical complement pathway** and the **alternative complement pathway**.

Molecules of the classical pathway are designated **C1, C2, C3** etc., whilst those of the alternative pathway are identified by letters, e.g. **factor B, factor D**.

The components of the complement systems interact with each other in a sequential manner such that the product of one reaction forms the enzyme for the next. This leads to the formation of an enzyme complex which binds and cleaves C3 — the third component of the complement cascade. This component is central to both pathways and forms the point at which the paths converge. Subsequent components and complexes act to form the membrane attack complex (MAC), which ultimately causes lysis of the cell/micro-organism on which it forms.

Cleavage fragments of complement molecules are identified by an appropriate subscript. Classically, the small fragments have been denoted by 'a' (e.g. C3a, C5a) and the large fragments by 'b' (e.g. C3b, C5b). Unfortunately, the fragments of C2 do not follow this notation; the larger fragment is designated 'a' and the smaller fragment 'b'.

Complement components with active enzyme sites are indicated by the presence of a bar over the top.

The Classical Complement Pathway

The classical complement pathway is normally activated by IgG or IgM containing immune complexes (antibody bound to specific antigen) which bind to the first component, C1. In addition, the acute-phase protein C reactive protein, endotoxins and some viruses may activate the classical pathway.

C1

C1 comprises three different types of molecule — C1q, C1r and C1s — which, in the presence of calcium, are held together (Figure 5.1). The Fc portion of an antibody in an immune complex binds to the globular heads of the six subunits which comprise C1q. The affinity of C1q for immunoglobulin alone is very weak but when several Fc regions are aggregated together (as in an immune complex), the affinity of the binding is greatly increased. Not all forms of immunoglobulin bind to C1 with the same affinity; some classes are better than others at activating the classical complement pathway (Table 5.1).

The enzymatic activity of C1 resides in the C1r and C1s chains. Each molecule of C1 comprises one molecule of C1q and two molecules each of C1r and C1s. Binding of antibody to C1q leads to the cleavage of the two chains of C1r, which in turn cleaves the C1s chains into long and short fragments. This results in the appearance of an enzymatic site on C1s which acts on the next component in the pathway — C4.

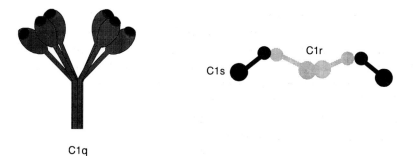

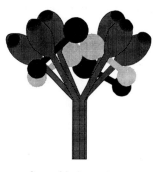

Assembled complex

Figure 5.1 Representation of the structure of the first component of the complement cascade.

C1q comprises six subunits with globular heads and associates with two molecules each of C1s and C1r

Table 5.1 Effectiveness of different classes of antibody in classical pathway activation

Class	Subclass	Classical pathway
IgM		+ + + +
IgG		
	IgG$_1$	+ + + +
	IgG$_2$	+
	IgG$_3$	+ + +
	IgG$_4$	—
IgA		—
IgE		—
IgD		—

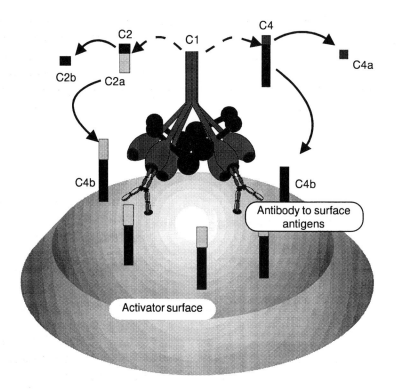

Figure 5.2 Formation of the classical pathway C3 convertase.
C1 is activated by immune complexes and splits C4 and C2. C4b binds the activator surface and C2a to form the C3 convertase. C4a and C2b are soluble fragments with other biological properties

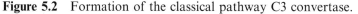

C4

C4 has three chains, the largest of which—the α chain—is cleaved by C1s, causing the release of a small fragment—C4a. The larger fragment—C4b—binds to the target antigen via the formation of covalent amide or ester bonds. In the presence of magnesium ions, C4b bound to the target antigen is capable of interacting with, and binding, the next component of complement—C2.

C2

C2 is a single-chain molecule which binds to C4b and, in the presence of C1s, is cleaved. The larger fragment—C2a—contains the enzymatic site of the C2 molecule and remains in the complex, whilst the smaller fragment is released. This new complex—C4b2a—acquires the ability to activate the next component in the classical pathway, C3. This complex is also known as the **classical pathway C3 convertase** (Figure 5.2).

Both C4b and C2a have labile active sites and most of the molecules formed lose their binding sites before achieving association with membranes or one another, diffusing away as inactive reaction products. C4b2a is unstable and decays, losing the C2 peptide (from its binding site on C4b) as an enzymatically inactive fragment. C4b bound to an activator can accept another molecule of C2 and, in the presence of active C1, will form an active enzyme capable of continuing the complement cascade.

C3

C3 has two disulphide-linked chains (α and β) and, like C4, has an internal thiolester bond in the α chain. When this bond is cleaved, the molecule undergoes a conformational change which leads to an alteration in its biochemical properties.

When C4b2a acts on C3, a small peptide is cleaved from the α chain — C3a. This exposes a thiolester bond in the remaining fragment — C3b — which will interact with any suitable acceptor in the environment (e.g. molecules with exposed reactive hydroxyl or amino groups). If this thiolester bond does not form a covalent bond with an appropriate acceptor, it is hydrolysed through interaction with water in the tissues. The majority of cleaved C3 molecules fail to bind to an activator (e.g. cell membranes, micro-organisms).

The attachment of C3b to membranes leads to the formation of C4b2a3b, which is covalently bound to the antigen (via the C3 thiolester linkage) and forms the **classical pathway C5 convertase** (Figure 5.3). This cleaves C5 into two fragments — C5a and C5b — the larger of which — C5b — associates with the convertase and can interact with subsequent components of the complement cascade, leading to lysis of membranes and micro-organisms.

The smaller fragments released by the actions of the enzymes of the classical complement pathway — i.e. C3a, C4a and C5a — have a number of potent biological effects which are important in inflammation and will be discussed later.

The Alternative Complement Pathway

In the alternative complement pathway, C3 exists in two molecular forms: the native form which circulates in the serum, and a conformationally altered form in which the thiolester bond has been hydrolysed. This altered C3 can bind another factor in the presence of magnesium ions — factor B of the alternative pathway. In the presence of factor D (a serine protease), factor B may be cleaved to form Bb. These proteins are analogous to the C4b, C2 and C1 of the classical pathway respectively. Together they form the **alternative pathway C3 convertase — C3bBb** (Figure 5.4). Like the convertase of the classical pathway, it catalyses the breakdown of C3 to C3a and C3b. The C3b so formed may

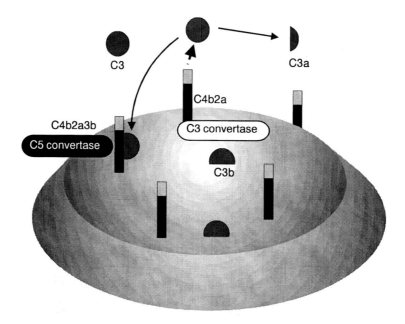

Figure 5.3   Formation of the classical pathway C5 convertase.
The C3 convertase attached to the activator splits C3, the larger fragment of which (C3b) attaches to the activator, leading to the formation of C4b2a3b, which is covalently bound to the antigen and forms the classical pathway C5 convertase

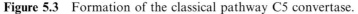

either continue the alternative pathway activation by binding factor B, or it may bind the C3 convertase to form the **alternative pathway C5 convertase**—**(C3b)$_n$Bb**. This compound is extremely unstable under normal physiological conditions and is stabilised by another serum protein—**properdin (C3b$_n$PBb)**.

Activation of the alternative pathway may be achieved through the presence of surfaces to which the conformationally altered C3 may attach, e.g. rabbit erythrocytes, Gram-negative bacteria, aggregates of IgA and certain B lymphocytes. Once attached, the alternative pathway C3 convertase becomes highly active and is able to act on large numbers of C3 molecules to produce C3a and C3b. Like the classical pathway, the alternative pathway may be activated by immune complexes, IgA-containing complexes being the most efficient (Table 5.2).

The Membrane Attack Complex

The **membrane attack complex (MAC)** is formed by complement components C5 to C9. Upon attachment to its convertase (derived from either the classical or alternative pathways), C5 is cleaved into C5a and C5b. The latter binds to its ligand—C6. Failure to do so results in its swift inactivation. The C5b6 complex so formed binds C7; the resulting complex, being relatively hydrophobic,

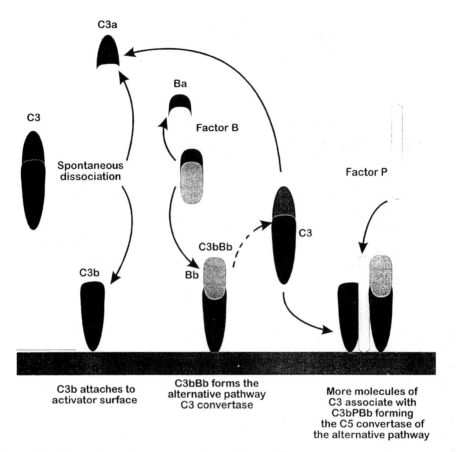

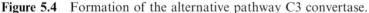

Figure 5.4   Formation of the alternative pathway C3 convertase.
  C3 can naturally exist in an altered form which can bind factor B of the alternative pathway. In the presence of factor D (a serine protease), factor B may be cleaved to form Bb. These proteins are analogous to the C4b, C2 and C1 of the classical pathway respectively. Together they form the alternative pathway C3 convertase—C3bBb

interacts with lipids present in the membranes surrounding the immunogen (Figure 5.5).
  The C7 molecule, when bound to the C5b6 complex, can insert in the membrane and may bind a single molecule of C8. The resulting small, highly charged channel is stabilised by the incorporation of several molecules of C9, giving rise to a cylindrical, pore-like structure which spans the membrane (Figure 5.6). The stability of this membrane attack complex (MAC)— $C5b678(9)_n$—arises from the association between the hydrophobic exterior of the MAC with membrane lipids. The hydrophilic interior of the channel allows the loss of water and small ions from the target cell, thus eliminating its osmotic and chemical balance and resulting in lysis (Figure 5.7).

Table 5.2   Effectiveness of different classes of antibody in alternative pathway activation

Class	Subclass	Alternative pathway
IgM		+ +
IgG		
	IgG$_1$	+ +
	IgG$_2$	+ +
	IgG$_3$	+ +
	IgG$_4$	+ +
IgA		+ + +
IgE		+ +
IgD		+ +

Regulation of Complement Activation

Since the formation of the MAC is antigen-independent and it may attach to cell surfaces in the vicinity and cause lysis of nearby host cells, it is vital to maintain strict control of the complement system. It has powerful lytic and inflammatory activities and, if uncontrolled, may lead to serious tissue damage.

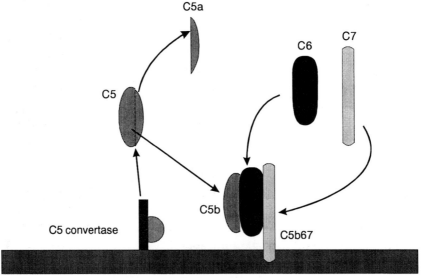

Figure 5.5   Formation of the C5b67 complex.

The C5 convertase splits C5, allowing the fragment C5b to attach to the antigen. This binds to C6, and the C5b6 complex so formed binds C7. This complex is relatively hydrophobic and interacts with lipids present in the membranes surrounding the antigen

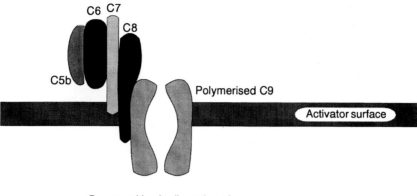

C6 C7
C8
C5b
Polymerised C9
Activator surface

Pore resulting in disruption of
activator

Figure 5.6 Formation of the membrane attack complex.

The C7 molecule, when bound to the C5b6 complex, can insert in the membrane and may bind a single molecule of C8. The resulting small, highly charged channel is stabilised by the incorporation of several molecules of C9, giving rise to a cylindrical, pore-like structure which causes lysis of the cell

Neither the classical, nor the alternative, pathway can be activated by antibody alone; it must be bound to antigen to be effective. In addition, a single antibody molecule bound to antigen is ineffectual; more than one must coat the antigen before complement can be activated. This limitation is probably an important method of regulation, since relatively large amounts of specific antibody must be formed before complement activation can occur. Infections which are controlled quickly and effectively by other mechanisms may only stimulate a small antibody response. If the organism has already been eliminated, activation of complement would probably lead to pathology (tissue damage). By contrast, a poorly controlled infection with increasing micro-organismal load will stimulate a strong antibody response, leading to complement activation which may help to eliminate the infecting agent.

Regulation is achieved at different stages of complement activation through the involvement of other proteins. The **C1 inhibitor (C1INH)** prevents the function of activated C1s and C1r by binding to their active sites. It also inhibits activated Hageman factor (one of the components of the clotting cascade) and all the systems activated by Hageman factor fragments. Thus, C1INH regulates enzymes of the kinin-generating system (chemicals which stimulate the sensation of pain), the clotting system and the fibrinolytic system (molecules involved in the regulation of blood clotting and wound repair). The importance of this regulatory protein in prevention of pathological damage is evidenced by the immunodeficiency disease hereditary angioneurotic oedema (HANE), where sufferers are unable to produce normal levels of functional C1INH. This is discussed further in Chapter 16.

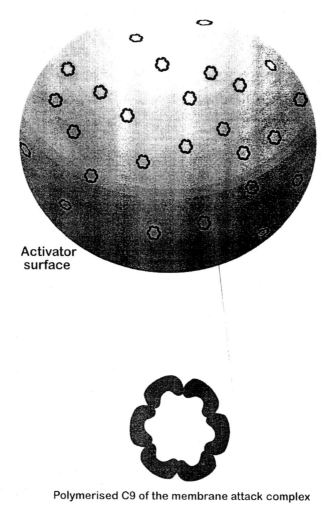

Polymerised C9 of the membrane attack complex

Figure 5.7   Structure of the pores formed by the membrane attack complex.
   The polymerised C9 forms pore-like structures in the target cell membrane, resulting in osmotic imbalance and cellular lysis

C4-binding protein (C4BP) and **factor I** (which is a protease) regulate the action of C4b. Factor I may cleave (and therefore inactivate) C4b once it is attached to its binding protein. Factor I, in the presence of factor H, may also cleave the α chain of hydrolysed C3 or C3b in two places to form a partially degraded molecule — iC3b. This molecule does not play a part in the complement cascade but is capable of promoting phagocytosis. In addition, under appropriate conditions, Factor I can degrade iC3b further to C3dg. Regulation by factors I and H is dependent upon the surface to which C3b is bound. If the surface is that of a micro-organism, the C3b is protected from factors H and I, which are unable to bind, and the complement cascade proceeds to its termination with the formation of the MAC. By contrast, when C3b is bound to host cell membranes, factors H and I are able to interact with it, causing its degradation and preventing the continuation of the pathway. This difference in ability to bind to certain surfaces appears to be related to the presence of charged carbohydrates such as sialic acid on mammalian cells which promote the binding of factor H.

Regulation of the MAC formation also occurs. Vibronectin (S protein) binds to C5b67 complexes and prevents their binding to cell membranes. Although C8 and C9 can still bind to the complex in the fluid phase, it cannot insert into membranes and cause lysis.

INFLAMMATION

Inflammation is the body's reaction to an injury such as invasion by a micro-organism or mechanical or chemical damage. The response may be initiated by the release of chemicals from damaged tissue cells either as a direct response to trauma or as a result of factors released from micro-organisms such as toxins. However, it is difficult to define precisely what triggers the inflammatory response, since it involves a large number of different cells and mediators. All the events which occur in inflammation are geared towards increasing the local blood flow (caused by dilation of the blood vessels) and the permeability of the vasculature (blood vessels). This allows cells and serum components increased access to the area of tissue damage in order to limit spread of infection and tissue damage and to promote healing. This increased permeability leads to the five cardinal signs of inflammation — heat, redness, pain, swelling and loss of function.

The inflammatory process involves the concerted action of the immune, kinin, fibrinolytic and clotting systems, which interact to maintain the integrity of the vascular system and to limit the spread of infection/damage. Figure 5.8 illustrates the complexity of the interaction between the components of the inflammatory response. The following sections will describe some of the chemicals and cellular functions involved in inflammation.

Inflammatory Mediators

Toxins from micro-organisms and enzymes released from the lysosomes of polymorphs cause or enhance tissue damage through the release of a number of chemicals from a variety of cells. Amongst these are the **prostaglandins (PGs)** and **leukotrienes (LTs)**, which belong to a family of unsaturated fatty acids derived from **arachidonic acid**, which is a component of most cell membranes. The different molecules have different effects but in general they are responsible for the induction of pain, fever, vascular permeability and chemotaxis (directed migration) of polymorphonuclear leukocytes (Table 5.3). Although mast cells

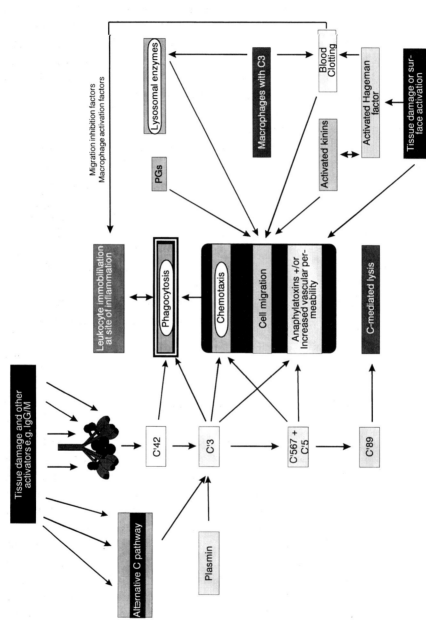

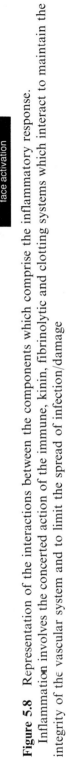

Figure 5.8 Representation of the interactions between the components which comprise the inflammatory response. Inflammation involves the concerted action of the immune, kinin, fibrinolytic and clotting systems which interact to maintain the integrity of the vascular system and to limit the spread of infection/damage

and basophils are the principal producers of these inflammatory mediators, other cells such as eosinophils, neutrophils and platelets are also capable of doing so.

Substances released as a result of tissue damage may activate mast cells. Their degranulation results in the release of **vasoactive amines** such as **histamine**. In addition, basophils and platelets release both histamine and **serotonin (5-hydroxytryptamine)**. These mediators cause increased capillary permeability. They are also important in the repair of tissue damage, as demonstrated in patients treated with large doses of antihistamines. Such individuals showed considerable impairment in the healing of surgical wounds. Indeed, evidence suggests that histamine (and perhaps other inflammatory mediators) may play a role in normal growth — especially fetal growth.

When tissue injury occurs, enzymes are released and surfaces are exposed which cause the activation of Hageman factor XII of the clotting cascade. This in turn activates, and is activated by, factor XI of the clotting cascade and kallikrein of the kinin system. The kinin system (a series of serum peptides which are sequentially activated) produces **bradykinin**, which causes pain, vasodilation and increased capillary permeability. This allows cells and serum proteins such as components of the complement cascade to pass into the tissues at the site of injury. If micro-organisms are present at the site, the complement cascade may be activated and complement fragments, particularly C3a and C5a, are released. These have dramatic, pro-inflammatory effects which are summarised in Table 5.4. Indeed, studies in complement-deficient animal models have suggested that complement activation is vital for the development of acute inflammation.

Cellular Responses in Inflammation

As a result of the action of inflammatory mediators, the flow of cells within the blood vessels slows, the cells becoming located along the walls of the vessel. The mediators also affect the expression of certain molecules on the endothelial cells lining the capillaries. These molecules promote the adherence of white blood cells (which express the corresponding receptor molecules), allowing them to move over the surface of the vessel wall in a process known as **pavementing**. The cells extend pseudopodia between the endothelial cells and secrete chemicals to dissolve the basement membrane, allowing them to squeeze out of the capillaries into the tissues. This migration is known as **diapedesis**.

Once in the tissues, cells detect certain molecules which have diffused away from the site of infection/damage and move to that site by a process known as **chemotaxis**. The diffusion of these **chemotaxins** follows the laws of chemistry (the molecules moving from a site of high concentration to one of low concentration), thus establishing a gradient which the cells are thought to detect via surface receptors. One explanation proposed for the movement of cells up

Table 5.3 Characteristics of some chemical mediators of inflammation

Substance	Chemistry	Produced by/from	Characteristics/functions
Heparin	Proteoglycan	Degranulation of mast cells	It is an anticoagulant, i.e. it prevents blood clotting. It temporarily suspends blood clotting, allowing inflammatory cells to enter the area of tissue injury
Histamine	Vasoactive amine	Mast cells and basophils, where it is stored in cytoplasmic granules	Released upon degranulation caused by cross-linking of surface Fc receptors. Acts on the endothelial cells of the blood vessels, causing them to become less tightly associated. This makes the blood vessels 'leaky' and allows inflammatory cells and serum proteins, such as antibody and complement components, to enter the area of tissue damage. Also causes the contraction of bronchiolar and vascular smooth muscle and increased secretion by nasal and bronchial mucous glands. Its effects are maximal after 1–2 minutes and last for about 10 minutes
Serotonin (5-hydroxytryptamine)	Derived from tryptophan	Granules of human platelets, whence it is released during the process of blood clotting	It is a neurotransmitter in the central nervous system. Its ability to cause leakage from the blood vessels derives from its effect on the endothelial cells, which become partially detached from each other
Kinins	Small basic peptides	The kallikreins (arginine esterases) act on kininogens (large proteins present in the plasma) to give kinins	Affect the movement of smooth muscle, increase vascular permeability and vasodilation and induce pain. Bradykinin is a 9 amino acid peptide derived from a serum α_2-macroglobulin precursor. It causes slow, sustained contraction of smooth muscles, including those of the bronchi and vessels, increased vascular permeability, increased secretion by mucous glands, including those of the bronchi, and stimulation of pain fibres. It also activates phospholipase A_2, which stimulates arachidonic acid metabolism

Eosinophil chemo-tactic factors	Tetrapeptides	Mast cell granules	Attract eosinophils to the site of inflammation and may play a role in activation of the cells
Prostaglandins and thromboxanes	Derived by cyclo-oxygenase metabolism of arachidonic acid	Lung mast cells. Neutrophils, macrophages	Human lung mast cells preferentially form PGD_2, a potent vasodilator. From neutrophils and macrophages, this pathway generates PGF_{2a}, a potent bronchoconstrictor, and PGE_1 and PGE_2, potent broncho- and vasodilators that regulate the tissue microenvironment. PGI_2 causes disaggregation of platelets, while thromboxanes (TXA_2 and TXB_2) aggregate platelets and thus are potent regulators of blood coagulation and homeostasis
Leukotrienes	Metabolites of arachidonic acid	Antigen–antibody interactions; neutrophils	Leukotrienes are potent spasmogenic and vasodilatory lipoxy-genases chiefly involved in the continued bronchospasm of asthma. Also known as slow-reacting substance of anaphylaxis (LTC_4, LTD_4, LTE_4). 5-Lipoxygenase generates 5-hydroxyeico-satetraenoic acid (5-HETE) which modulates cell motility and possibly glucose transport, and LTB_4, which is a potent chemotactic agent comparable to C5a.
Platelet-activating factors	Compounds derived from glycerol	IgE-containing ICs and by non-IgE reactions from basophils and alveolar macrophages	Released from platelets, granulocytes, monocytes, macrophages, mast cells and endothelial cells. Very potent, it causes activation of neutrophils and monocytes, causing the release of inflammatory mediators; induces lymphocyte proliferation and IL-2 secretion; platelet aggregation and thromboxane release

Table 5.4   The role of complement activation in inflammation

Proteins	Product of activation	Activity
C3, C4, C5	C3a, C4a, C5a	Anaphylatoxins which have intense effects on muscles and blood flow. At its worst extreme, anaphylaxis may result in death. Cause smooth muscle contraction, and degranulation of mast cells and basophils leading to release of histamine and other vasoactive substances that induce capillary leakage. C5a is the most potent anaphylatoxin
C3, C5	C3a, C5a	C3a and C5a have important immunoregulatory effects on T cell function, either stimulating (C5a) or inhibiting (C3a) aspects of cell-mediated immunity
C5	C5a	C5a is a potent chemotactic agent for neutrophils and monocytes. It increases neutrophil adherence and causes aggregation, stimulates neutrophil oxidative metabolism and the production of toxic oxygen species, and triggers lysosomal enzyme release from phagocytes

the gradient suggests that engagement of these receptors on a particular area of the cell surface stimulates pseudopod formation in that area and hence movement. As the concentration increases, more of the receptors are engaged over a wider surface, and, at the top of the gradient, enough of the surface receptors are engaged to prevent movement in any one direction. A number of molecules can act as chemotactic agents, including C3a and C5a as well as a group of cytokines known as **chemokines** (Table 5.5). This is a large family of structurally and functionally related pro-inflammatory molecules which stimulate the migration and activation of a variety of cells, including neutrophils, monocytes, lymphocytes and fibroblasts. Both neutrophils and monocytes are attracted by C5a but neutrophils predominate in acute inflammation, due to their larger number in the circulation. Once cells have reached the site of tissue injury, they are capable of phagocytosing any debris or pathogens which may be present.

Phagocytosis

The process of phagocytosis may be divided into a number of sequential stages: **opsonisation**, **ingestion** and **digestion**; we shall discuss each of these in turn. Although tissue macrophages are often the first cells to encounter and ingest an invading micro-organism, they are not very efficient at killing. This is best achieved by neutrophils, which may be attracted to the site of infection as a result of mediators released by macrophages. Neutrophils are by far the most

Table 5.5 Some characteristics of chemokines

Chemokine		Description
Interleukin-8	Major cellular sources	Produced by many cells, including monocytes, lymphocytes, granulocytes, fibroblasts, endothelial cells, hepatocytes, keratinocytes
	Major inducers	IL-1 and tumour necrosis factor
	Effects	Inflammatory cytokine which acts as a neutrophil and T cell chemoattractive and activating factor. It also attracts basophils and a subpopulation of lymphocytes. It is a potent angiogenic factor.
Macrophage inflammatory proteins 1α and 1β	Major cellular sources	Monocytes/macrophages, T cells and B cells
	Major inducers	Lipopolysaccharide (LPS; monocytes and macrophages), antibody to CD3 or phytohaemagglutinin (PHA) and phorbol myristate acetate (T cells), *S. aureus* Cowan strain (B cells)
	Effects	In vitro, stimulates chemokinesis and H_2O_2 production by neutrophils (human); acts as a prostaglandin-independent endogenous pyrogen (rabbit); MIP-1α is a stem cell inhibitor (mouse), an activity that may be antagonised by MIP-1β
Monocyte chemo-attractant protein	Major cellular sources	PHA-stimulated peripheral blood mononuclear cells, fibroblasts, endothelial cells, certain tumour cells and monocytes
	Major inducers	Some cells (e.g. certain tumour cells) express it constitutively; endothelial cells produce it after IL-1, TNF or LPS stimulation. Conflicting evidence exists over the production by monocytes, i.e. whether it is constitutive or induced
	Effects	Monocyte chemotaxis; enhances monocyte killing of certain tumour cell lines
RANTES	Major cellular sources	T lymphocytes
	Major inducers	May be constitutively expressed and enhanced on stimulation with Ag or PHA
	Effects	Chemoattractant for monocytes and T cells. Shows subset specificity, and migrating T cells are particularly enriched for CD4+ cells bearing markers which are thought to identify memory cells

efficient of the professional phagocytes. However, newly recruited macrophages (derived from blood monocytes attracted to the site of infection) also show the ability to kill phagocytosed organisms. Eosinophils, which are also efficient killers, are geared to killing extracellular pathogens which are too large to phagocytose, such as parasites like *Schistosoma* spp.

Opsonisation.   Once at the site of inflammation, phagocytes have to recognise the causative agent. They have a number of receptors which non-specifically attach to a variety of micro-organisms. This attachment is enhanced by **opsonins**.

OPSONIN

This is something which coats a particle and makes it more easy to phagocytose. For example, complement activation at the site of inflammation causes C3b to be deposited on the causative agent (which may be a micro-organism or an inert particle). Both neutrophils and macrophages have receptors for C3b which allows them to recognise their targets.

There are three main types of opsonin: **IgG antibodies**, **fragments of the complement protein C3** and **certain carbohydrates (CHO)** or **CHO-binding proteins**. Each may act as a 'go-between', binding the particle at one site and a specific receptor molecule on the surface of the phagocyte at the other end. The receptors for IgG (FcγR) and those binding CHO or CHO-binding proteins are always in an active state and stimulate ingestion immediately following ligand–receptor interaction. By contrast, the C3-fragment receptors (Table 5.6) are inactive and require a further signal in the form of a lymphokine, fibronectin or an acute-phase protein before activation may occur. Acute-phase proteins— such as C reactive protein (CRP)—can bind to the surface of micro-organisms and, having structures similar to C1, activate the classical complement pathway, leading to opsonisation by complement.

Ingestion.   The process of taking extracellular material into a cell is known as **endocytosis**. The active uptake of particulate material through the formation of

Table 5.6   Complement receptors involved in opsonisation

Receptor	Ligands
CR1	C3b
CR2	C3dg > C3d > iC3b > C3b

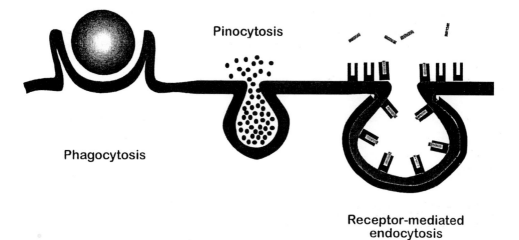

Pinocytosis

Phagocytosis

Receptor-mediated
endocytosis

Figure 5.9   Illustration of the different methods for uptake of extracellular material.
The process of taking extracellular material into a cell is known as endocytosis. The active uptake of particulate material through the formation of pseudopodia is known as phagocytosis. Pinocytosis is the process by which cells take up soluble material

pseudopodia is known as **phagocytosis**. **Pinocytosis** is the process by which cells take up soluble material (Figure 5.9).

When a particle attaches to a phagocyte (either non-specifically through chemical attraction or specifically through immunoglobulin or complement receptors), it stimulates the cell membrane which, as a result, forms pseudopodia or finger-like projections which surround the particle. They ultimately fuse together, engulfing the particle in a membrane-bound vesicle known as a **phagosome**. This is thought to be achieved by the transformation of the fluid cytoplasm (cytosol) into a gel by interaction with actin-binding proteins located on the inner surface of the cell membrane. This gelation results from the polymerisation of actin in the cytoplasm to form filaments which connect with each other and myosin, giving a more rigid gel-like consistency, and is stimulated by the activation signal received as a result of the occupancy of an opsonin receptor. The activated actin transmits a signal to the **myosin**, which contracts; this leads to the streaming of the cytosol, which pushes the plasma membrane in one direction, thus forming the pseudopod (Figure 5.10).

The precise details of how engulfment is initiated are not fully understood. It is thought that receptor occupancy by an opsonin (or micro-organism) results in signals which cause changes in the cytoplasm leading to the release of oxidising agents such as hydrogen peroxide which oxidise the sulphydryl groups of membrane proteins. This leads to intermolecular disulphide bonds linking adjacent receptors. This proceeds as the pseudopod advances around the particle, with receptors binding ligands rather like a zip (Figure 5.11).

Once formed, the phagosome moves to the interior of the cell, where degradation of its contents occurs.

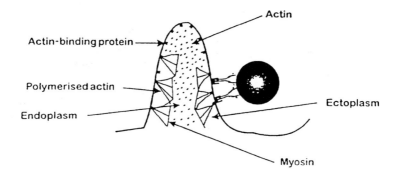

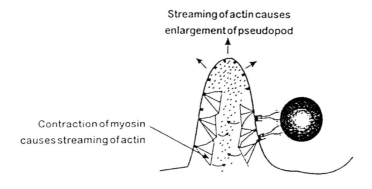

Figure 5.10 Intracellular processes leading to pseudopodia formation.

Pseudopodium formation is thought to occur due to the transformation of the fluid cytoplasm (cytosol) into a gel by interaction with actin-binding proteins located on the inner surface of the cell membrane. This gelation results from the polymerisation of actin in the cytoplasm to form filaments which connect with each other and myosin, giving a more rigid, gel-like consistency. The activated actin transmits a signal to the myosin, which contracts, leading to the streaming of the cytosol, pushing the plasma membrane in one direction, thus forming the pseudopod

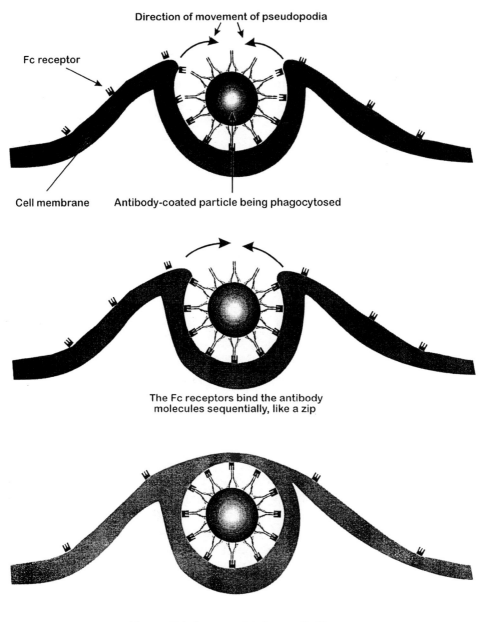

Direction of movement of pseudopodia

Fc receptor

Cell membrane   **Antibody-coated particle being phagocytosed**

The Fc receptors bind the antibody
molecules sequentially, like a zip

The particle becomes totally engulfed in
a phagosome

Figure 5.11   The 'zipper' method of receptor-mediated endocytosis.

Receptor occupancy by an opsonin (or micro-organism) is thought to result in the production of signals which cause changes in the cytoplasm leading to the release of oxidising agents such as hydrogen peroxide, which oxidise the sulphydryl groups of membrane proteins. This leads to intermolecular disulphide bonds linking adjacent receptors. This proceeds as the pseudopod advances around the particle, with receptors binding ligands rather like a zip

Digestion.   Digestion of the phagosomal contents is achieved by a variety of enzymes which are introduced into the phagosome when cytoplasmic granules (polymorphs) and lysosomes (polymorphs and mononuclear phagocytes) empty their contents into the phagosome. These membrane-bound organelles fuse with the phagosomal membrane, forming a larger **phagolysosome**. This fusion may start before the phagosome is closed, and destructive enzymes may therefore be released outside the cell, resulting in the tissue damage associated with some immunological reactions.

One of the first events, which occurs immediately after ingestion, is the **acidification** of the phagosome. This starts before the granule contents are released and is caused by the accumulation of lactic acid and hydrogen ions produced by the respiratory burst. The hydrogen ions are actively moved into the lysosomes by special pumps which derive their energy from adenosine triphosphate (ATP). The pH rapidly reduces to about 4, assisted by the release of the acidic granule contents. Few micro-organisms can survive or multiply in an acid environment, and the lysosomal enzymes which bring about their destruction are most efficient at a low pH.

Once the contents of the phagolysosome have been destroyed, the debris must be eliminated. Some products of degradation may be re-used, such as amino acids, nucleotides, sugars and lipids. Other, more indigestible, parts may be exocytosed (although this is undesirable, since tissue-damaging enzymes are released at the same time), or may be stored within the cell until it dies and is eliminated from the body, e.g. in the faeces or sputum.

The Respiratory Burst

Upon stimulation, the phagocyte undergoes a respiratory burst (also known as the **oxidative** or **metabolic burst**) which is characterised by a rapid, marked increase in the consumption of oxygen by the cell and results in the production of **toxic oxygen metabolites**. Normally, respiration is mediated by mitochondrial enzymes. However, the respiratory burst involves the action of a group of enzymes which is known as the **nicotinamide adenine diphosphate oxidase (NADPH-oxidase)** found in the cytoplasm and associated with the membrane of the phagosome. The principal effect of this group of enzymes is to convert molecular oxygen to the superoxide anion—a highly reactive molecule which has two unpaired electrons, each available for association with another electron. Addition of one electron leads to the formation of superoxide; a second electron converts it to peroxide (Figure 5.12). This conversion is mediated by the reduced form of NADP—NADPH—which has an additional hydrogen atom attached to the nicotinamide ring and an extra electron associated with it. All these molecules with unpaired electrons are called **free radicals**. They are highly unstable and are capable of damaging proteins, lipids, DNA and cell membranes. Thus, they may be responsible for the destruction of phagocytosed

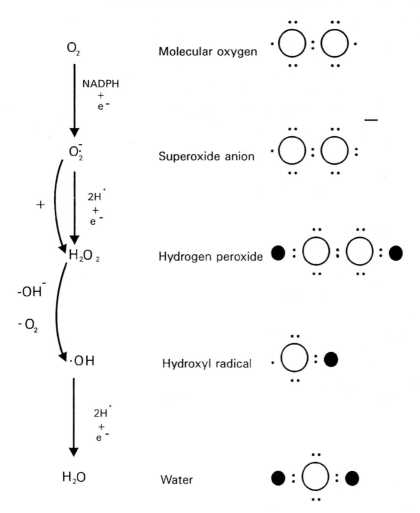

Figure 5.12   Conversion of molecular oxygen to reactive intermediates.

The respiratory burst involves the action of a group of enzymes known as the nicotinamide adenine diphosphate oxidase (NADPH-oxidase). These enzymes convert molecular oxygen to the superoxide anion—a highly reactive molecule which has two unpaired electrons, each available for association with another electron. Addition of one electron leads to the formation of superoxide; a second electron converts it to peroxide

micro-organisms. Under normal circumstances, the free radicals and hydrogen peroxide are destroyed by endogenous scavenger enzymes. However, in activated phagocytes they are produced in greater quantities than can be destroyed, allowing them to accumulate and, indeed, to be secreted by the cells. Although the hydroxyl radicals are extremely short-lived, the superoxide and hydrogen peroxide are released in the tissues; their persistence (and hence the degree of resulting tissue damage) depends on the ability of the cells in the

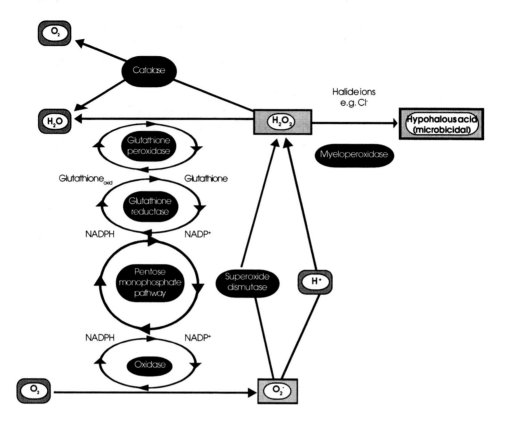

Figure 5.13 The production of toxic oxygen metabolites and other microbicidal compounds during the oxidative burst

locality to destroy them. Superoxide is acted on by **superoxide dismutase**, which converts it to hydrogen peroxide. The latter can be inactivated by **catalase** or **peroxidases** such as **glutathione peroxides**. If these enzymes are not available, the superoxide radical and hydrogen peroxide combine to produce hydroxyl radicals. In addition to these toxic oxygen metabolites, other microbicidal compounds are generated during the oxidative burst, including hypohalous acids (Figure 5.13).

LEARNING OUTCOMES

Having studied this chapter you should have an understanding of the complex events which make up the inflammatory response. This includes the mechanism of action of both the classical and alternative complement pathways and the biological activities of some of the complement fragments produced. The cellular interactions in inflammation lead to the generation of pro-inflammatory compounds which enhance the response, containing and eliminating any infectious agents and repairing any tissue damage. Also, it is important to remember that these highly reactive reagents (including the products of the respiratory burst) may themselves cause tissue damage and thus the whole process must be carefully regulated.

In order to help understand the material you have studied, test yourself on Chapter 5 using the program which accompanies this text. Some of the questions may be based on information available in Further Reading.

Chapter 6

Adaptive Immunity

LEARNING OBJECTIVES

When the body is exposed to an antigen for the first time, a number of non-specific (or **innate**) mechanisms are brought into play to restrict its spread and the accompanying tissue damage. They do not require specific identification of the invader, merely the recognition that something foreign has entered the system. These mechanisms are very efficient and manage to prevent infection by many organisms. However, the latter have been particularly adept in evolving ways to avoid destruction by these non-specific defence systems, and as a result, the host has developed more complex immune mechanisms which specifically recognise the invader and invoke reactions to destroy it. This **adaptive immunity** is characterised by the development of both T and B lymphocyte memory cells, which allow a more rapid and effective response on second exposure to the eliciting antigen.

In this chapter we will look at all the mechanisms involved in adaptive immunity. This includes the processing and presentation of antigen, the development of specific T cell responses (with the associated lymphokine secretion) and the maturation of the antibody response (which involves the development of memory and switching of the class of antibody produced).

ANTIGEN-SPECIFIC IMMUNITY

The development of antigen-specific immunity largely depends on the ability of T cells to recognise antigen. This is a complex process, since T cells cannot bind free antigen and must have it presented to them by products of the **major histocompatibility gene complex** (**MHC**) on the membranes of accessory cells. T cells can only recognise antigen presented by self-MHC gene products.

In order for an antigen to associate with MHC gene products, it must be processed, because only short peptides may associate with the antigen-binding regions of these molecules (see Chapter 2).

Antigen Processing and Presentation

There are two major pathways of antigen processing and presentation which are not mutually exclusive but which depend partly on whether the antigen may be classified as endogenous or exogenous. In general, peptides from exogenous antigens associate with MHC Class II molecules and those from endogenous antigens with products of the MHC Class I genes.

When T cells recognise antigen, the T cell receptor (TCR)–MHC–antigen complex is further stabilised by interaction between the CD4 or CD8 molecule and the MHC molecule. Antigen presented by Class II gene products are recognised by T cells which express the CD4 antigen. These are responsible generally for initiating a protective immune response. Antigens presented by Class I gene products are recognised by T cells which express the CD8 antigen and which may be capable of lysing the cell expressing the antigen. This combination of Class II–CD4 and Class I–CD8 may be logically explained as shown in Figure 6.1.

Generation of Peptides Presented by MHC Class I Molecules

Most of the peptides presented by Class I molecules are derived from proteins present in the nucleus or the cytoplasm, although some have been shown to be derived from proteins in the mitochondria or endoplasmic reticulum (ER). In general, those peptides which associate with Class I molecules must be processed in the nucleus or cytoplasm by a highly controlled mechanism which allows only partial degradation and not complete reduction to constituent amino acids (Figure 6.2). This regulation is important, since it has been shown that the amino acids surrounding the epitope to be presented may influence the breakdown of a particular protein. However, currently, this is the limit of our knowledge about the specificity of this breakdown process, except that many of the proteins involved are degraded by a large, ATP-dependent, proteolytic complex called the **proteasome**.

Breakdown products produced in the cytoplasm are transferred to the lumen of the ER by the peptide transporters **TAP1** and **TAP2** (**T**ransporter **a**ssociated with **A**ntigen **P**resentation). Evidence suggests that these molecules show some specificity in the peptides they transport.

Once inside the ER, it is thought that the peptides may be modified further by local proteases which produce peptides of the correct size for binding to Class I molecules, the latter subsequently protecting these peptides from total degradation. Recent research has shown that only peptides 8–10 amino acids long can fit the binding groove of a Class I molecule, this length being restricted by the interaction between the amino and carboxyl termini of the peptide and the extremities of the groove. At specific defined positions, major amino acids have been identified in a number of different peptides obtained

A). Potential outcome if CD8 positive, cytotoxic T cells recognised antigen in association with MHC Class II

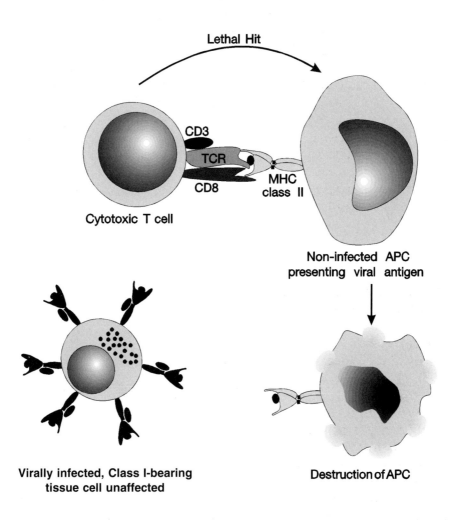

Lethal Hit

CD3

TCR

CD8

MHC class II

Cytotoxic T cell

Non-infected APC presenting viral antigen

Virally infected, Class I-bearing tissue cell unaffected

Destruction of APC

NON-PRODUCTIVE OUTCOME

Figure 6.1 Outcome of the interaction between MHC molecules and T cells during antigen presentation.

Any cell may be infected by a virus, and therefore the immune system must be able to recognise foreign antigen in association with MHC molecules on such cells, so that cytotoxic T cells can eliminate the infection. Since MHC Class I molecules are present on all nucleated cells, CD8 + T cells recognise antigen in association with MHC Class I (B). If they recognised antigen in association with MHC Class II molecules alone, then only antigen-presenting cells would be destroyed and the immune response would be eliminated (A)

B). Potential outcome when CD4 positive T cells recognise antigen in association with MHC Class II

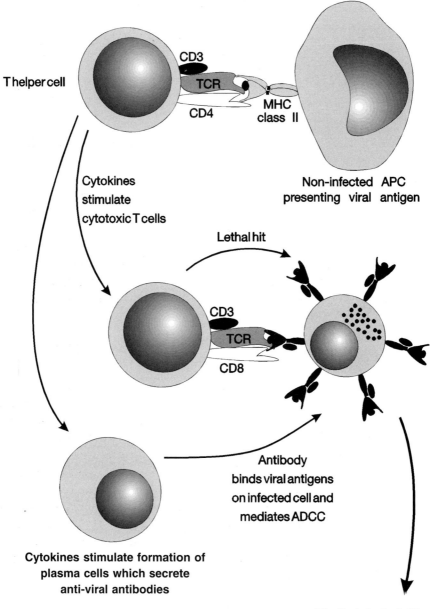

T helper cell

CD3

TCR

CD4

MHC class II

Non-infected APC presenting viral antigen

Cytokines stimulate cytotoxic T cells

Lethal hit

CD3

TCR

CD8

Antibody binds viral antigens on infected cell and mediates ADCC

Cytokines stimulate formation of plasma cells which secrete anti-viral antibodies

Virally infected, Class I-bearing tissue cell destroyed

PRODUCTIVE OUTCOME

from Class I molecules. These 'anchor residues' fit in pockets in the groove of a Class I molecule, thus dictating whether or not a particular peptide may bind to that molecule.

Assembly and Intracellular Transport of MHC Class I Molecules

Both the heavy and light chains of the MHC Class I molecules are synthesised in the ER. At physiological temperature, the Class I heterodimer is unstable but is stabilised by the association of presentable peptide. Other molecules, which transiently associate with the Class I heterodimer and are released upon binding of peptide, are thought to help Class I molecules achieve the correct folding upon synthesis.

In order for Class I-bound peptide to be presented on the cell surface, the heterotrimeric complex (Class I heavy chain, β_2-microglobulin and peptide) must be released from the ER. However, most Class I alleles only achieve limited assembly of the trimeric complex, which affects both the efficiency of the release and the rate of intracellular transport of the complex. Upon release from the ER, the Class I–peptide complexes are transported via the Golgi apparatus and the trans-Golgi reticulum to the cell surface. Class I (but not Class II) antigen processing can be inhibited by two agents; brefeldin A blocks movement of membrane proteins from the endoplasmic reticulum to the Golgi apparatus, and the adenovirus E3/19K gene product specifically binds to Class I molecules and retains them in the ER.

Generation of Peptides Presented by MHC Class II Molecules

The products of the MHC Class II genes are expressed on cells capable of endocytosis and present antigens derived from an extracellular source (Figure 6.3). After endocytosis, **endosome–lysosome fusion** occurs and degradation of the antigen begins. Initially, the tertiary structure of a protein is destroyed by the reduction of disulphide bonds, thus making it more accessible to other degradative enzymes, which include the **cathepsins B, D and E**. Fragments of an antigen, regardless of their degree of degradation, can bind to Class II molecules but require further processing by **endosomal proteases** to produce a minimal fragment which is protected from further degradation by the Class II molecule itself. Distinct peptides bind with different affinities to the same Class II molecule. However, whether peptide–Class II association and affinity is governed by the primary sequence of the peptide is, as yet, unknown.

Assembly and Intracellular Transport of MHC Class II Molecules

Class II molecules are structurally similar to Class I molecules. However, during assembly, they associate with a third molecule — the **invariant chain**. Thus, Class

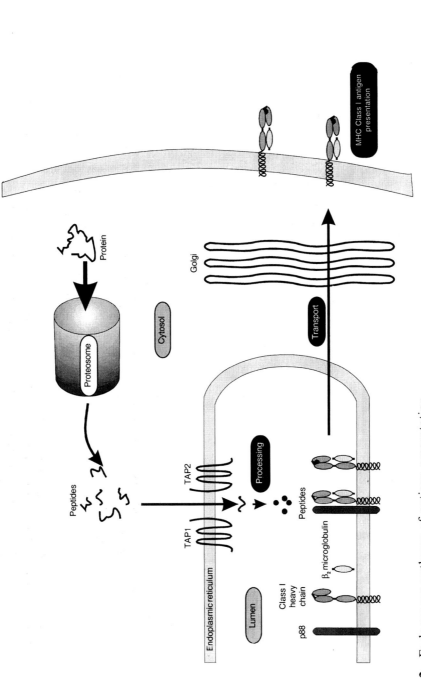

Figure 6.2 Endogenous pathway of antigen presentation.
Most of the peptides presented by Class I molecules are derived from proteins present in the nucleus or the cytoplasm, although some have been shown to be derived from proteins in the mitochondria or endoplasmic reticulum (ER). The peptide must be processed in the nucleus or cytoplasm by a highly controlled mechanism which allows only partial degradation and not complete reduction to constituent amino acids

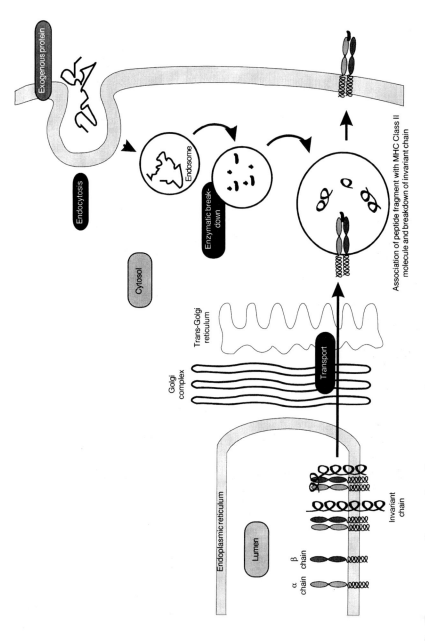

Figure 6.3 Exogenous pathway of antigen presentation.

The products of the MHC Class II genes are expressed on cells capable of endocytosis and present antigens derived from an extracellular source. Fragments of an antigen, regardless of their degree of degradation, can bind to Class II molecules but require further processing by endosomal proteases to produce a minimal fragment which is protected from further degradation by the Class II molecule itself

II molecules are assembled in the ER as a trimeric complex (composed of an α and β chain which present the antigen at the cell surface and the invariant chain).

Since Class II molecules are assembled in the ER like Class I molecules, they could, in theory, bind the same peptides. However, in vitro studies have shown that Class II molecules only bind peptide after removal of the invariant chain, which usually occurs beyond the ER. This suggests that the invariant chain may help to regulate peptide binding, although presentation of cytosolic or ER-derived peptides may occur.

The Class II-invariant chain trimers are exported in triplets. These **nonamers** are transported through the Golgi apparatus to the trans-Golgi reticulum, where signals derived from the cytoplasmic tail of the invariant chain direct them towards the endocytic pathway of antigen processing. Having entered this pathway, they remain there for up to 3 hours before appearing at the cell surface. Proteases (e.g. cathepsin B) digest the invariant chain, allowing processed peptides to bind to Class II molecules which are subsequently presented at the cell surface. Inhibition of this digestion (e.g. by **leupeptin**) prevents the expression of Class II molecules at the cell surface (as indeed do the lysosomotropic agents ammonium chloride and chloroquine).

ANTIGEN PRESENTATION IN ADAPTIVE IMMUNITY

T Cells

T cells show a wide range of responses to antigenic stimulation which may be influenced by a number of factors, including the type of antigen, the route of entry and the type of antigen-presenting cell, to name but a few. The outcome of such antigenic stimulation will depend partly on the type of T cell which predominates in the response, i.e. Th1 or Th2, and on whether antigen-specific memory cells are present. In addition, some effector T cells have the capability of directly eliminating cells via cytotoxic action. These activities represent the role of T cells in immunity, which is achieved by the secretion of chemical mediators known as cytokines.

T Cell Responses to Antigen Stimulation

T cells in the periphery may be considered to be either naive, memory or effector cells. **Naive cells** are those which have not been stimulated by antigen since leaving the thymus. By contrast, **memory cells** are those which have had antigen presented to them at least once and have returned to a resting state from which they can be activated on subsequent exposure to the same antigen. This group of cells are considered to be long-lived. However, individual cells within this group may be short-lived and persistence may depend upon restimulation by antigen. **Effector cells** are those T cells which, in response to presented antigen, are able to carry out specialised functions such as the secretion of specific cytokines or the lysis of target cells. These cells derive from either naive **or** memory cells several days after antigenic stimulation. They are short-lived, and in a highly activated state, but require further stimulation before they can perform their effector function. Studies in mice have shown that naive cells only secrete interleukin-2 (IL-2) on initial stimulation, whilst memory and effector cells may exhibit defined cytokine secretion profiles, e.g. Th1 and Th2 cell cytokine profiles. Recently, similar differential cytokine secretion profiles have been proposed for mouse CD8+ T cells.

When a host is exposed to an antigen, depending on the site of entry the antigen will be taken up by mononuclear phagocytes. However, antigen will also pass via the lymph to draining lymph nodes, where it will be taken up by other macrophages and dendritic cells. The latter have been clearly demonstrated to be most effective in presenting antigen to naive T cells, a process which occurs with great efficiency in lymph nodes, where T cells can enter from the blood or lymph and percolate through the antigen-presenting cell-rich tissues.

Interaction between a micro-organism and an antigen-presenting cell may lead to the production of certain cytokines. For example, the phagocytosis by macrophages of *Mycobacterium tuberculosis* stimulates the production of IL-12 (Table 6.1) by the macrophage, which encourages the subsequent development of a Th1 response. Depending on the nature of the pathogen involved, macrophages may be induced to produce IL-10 (Table 6.2), which stimulates a Th2 response, presumably through inhibiting the production of IL-12.

When a T cell recognises presented antigen, the interaction between the TCR–CD3–CD4 on the T cell and the antigen–MHC complex on the antigen-presenting cell results in a number of vital events which ultimately lead to activation of the T cell (summarised in Figure 6.4). Other molecules, which include CD28 (or CTLA4) on T cells and CD80 (a member of the family of molecules known as B7) on antigen-presenting cells, are vital for this activation, ensuring the correct signalling within the T cells. As a result of interaction with the T cell, the antigen-presenting cell is stimulated to secrete IL-1 (Table 6.3). This binds to IL-1 receptors on the T cell and augments the stimulatory signal from the early activation events. This results in the production of IL-2 and the expression of IL-2 receptors.

IL-2 is a polypeptide which is produced by, and acts on, T cells, promoting their proliferation (Table 6.4). It acts also on other cells of the immune system, such as natural killer (NK) and B cells. Cytokines exert their effects by binding specific receptors on the membrane of their target cells. There are three distinct receptors for IL-2 which differ in their affinity for the cytokine. The high-affinity receptor comprises three chains — the α, β and γ chains. The intermediate-affinity receptor comprises only the β and γ chains, whilst the low-affinity receptor is formed by the α chain alone. The IL-2 produced may act back on the cell which produced it (**autocrine effect**), enhancing its activation

Table 6.1   Characteristics of interleukin-12

Major cellular sources of IL-12	IL-12 is a heterodimer made up of two chains, p35 and p40, and is produced by B lymphoblastoid cells, monocytes/macrophages and B cells
Major inducers of IL-12	Micro-organisms, e.g. *Staphylococcus aureus*, *Mycobacterium tuberculosis*, *Toxoplasma gondii*, *Leishmania major* and the lipopolysaccharide from Gram-negative bacteria
Effects of IL-12	Important in defence against intracellular pathogens. Induces IFNγ production by T and NK cells; enhances NK and ADCC activity; co-stimulates peripheral blood lymphocyte proliferation; stimulates proliferation and induces the differentiation of Th1 cells
Cross-reactivity	Mouse IL-12 functions on human cells but **not** vice versa

Table 6.2   Characteristics of interleukin-10

Major cellular sources of IL-10	Th0 and Th2 subsets of murine T cells, activated CD4+ and CD8+ human T cells, murine Ly-1+ B cells, monocytes and macrophages
Effects of IL-10	Blocks activation of cytokine synthesis by Th1 T cells, activated monocytes and NK cells. Stimulates and/or enhances proliferation of B cells, thymocytes and mast cells and, with TGFβ, stimulates IgA production by human B cells
Cross-reactivity	Human IL-10 functions on murine cells but **not** vice versa

and proliferation, or it may diffuse away and affect other cells in the locality (paracrine effect). However, only those cells which have encountered antigen and thus are expressing IL-2 receptors are able to respond to this stimulus.

The interaction between IL-2 and its receptor initiates several intracellular signals which ultimately help to cause the proliferation and differentiation of distinct subsets of effector T cells.

Th0, Th1 and Th2 Cells

Subsets of T cells which have distinct patterns of cytokine production were described initially in mice. Although the distinction is not so clear-cut, it is now

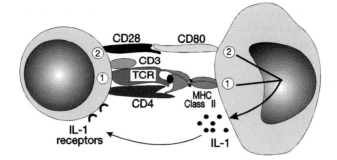

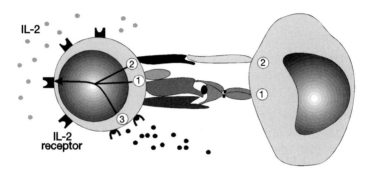

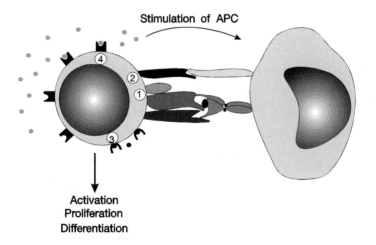

Figure 6.4 Molecular interactions leading to T cell activation.
When a T cell recognises presented antigen, the interaction between the TCR–CD3–CD4 on the T cell and the antigen–MHC complex on the antigen-presenting cell results in a number of vital events which ultimately lead to activation

Table 6.3 Characteristics of interleukin-1

Major cellular sources of IL-1	IL-1 is a polypeptide which exists in two forms — IL-1α and IL-1β. Both bind to the same receptor and have the same functions. IL-1 is synthesised as a large precursor molecule which is processed at the cell membrane or extracellularly to give the mature, active proteins. It is produced by many cells but most importantly monocytes, activated macrophages, dendritic cells, T and B cells, NK cells and LGLs. Mononuclear phagocytes produce mainly IL-1β
Major inducers of IL-1	Endotoxin, muramyl dipeptide; interaction with T cells during antigen presentation
Effects of IL-1	Induces fever, hypotension, neutrophilia and the acute-phase response in vivo
Cross-reactivity	Both human and mouse IL-1 have cross-species activity

Table 6.4 Characteristics of interleukin-2

Major cellular sources of IL-2	IL-2 is produced by T cells. A single disulphide bond between residues 58 and 105 of the molecule is essential to its biological activity
Receptors	The receptor for IL-2 exists in three forms: low, intermediate and high affinity. There are three constituent molecules, IL-2Rα, IL-2Rβ and IL-2Rγ chains, and differential expression of these molecules gives rise to the different affinity receptors, i.e. IL-2Rα alone binds IL-2 with low affinity, IL-2Rβ and IL-2Rγ bind with intermediate affinity, and IL-2Rα, IL-2Rβ and IL-2Rγ bind with high affinity. The α chain appears to be vital for the assembly of the high-affinity receptor, whilst the β chain is responsible for signalling to the cell that the receptor has been occupied, thus stimulating subsequent proliferation events. The γ chain helps stabilise the high-affinity receptor and helps in the cellular intake of IL-2
Effects of IL-2	Stimulates growth and differentiation of T, B, NK and LAK cells, monocytes, macrophages and oligo-dendrocytes
Cross-reactivity	Human IL-2 acts on mouse cells but **not** vice versa

generally accepted that these subsets—Th0, Th1 and Th2—do exist in humans. The cytokines produced by these subsets stimulate different types of immune response (Figure 6.5). Th1 cells produce cytokines which are responsible largely for the stimulation of cytotoxic effector cells and macrophage activities (known as cell-mediated immunity), i.e. IL-2, IFNγ (Table 6.5) and TNFα.

IFNγ has a variety of effects on B cells. It causes the preferential production of mIgG$_{2a}^+$ B cells, counteracts the effects of IL-4 on B cells and inhibits the proliferation of Th2 cells. By contrast, Th2 cells produce cytokines which promote the proliferation and differentiation of B lymphocytes, i.e. IL-4 (Table 6.6), IL-5 (Table 6.7), IL-6 (Table 6.8) and IL-13 (Table 6.9).

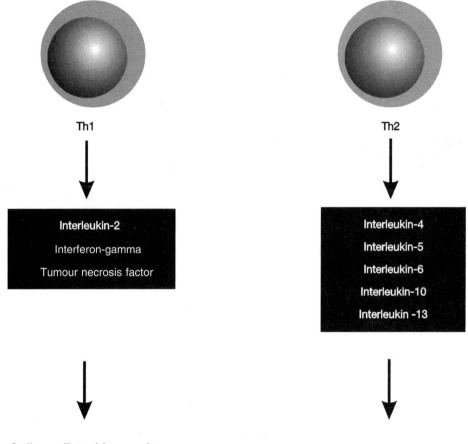

Figure 6.5 Cytokine secretion patterns of T helper subsets.

Subsets of T cells have different patterns of cytokine production which stimulate different types of immune response. Th1 cells produce cytokines which are responsible largely for the stimulation of cytotoxic effector cells and macrophage activities (known as cell-mediated immunity), i.e. IL-2, IFNγ, TNFα

Table 6.5 Characteristics of interferon-gamma

Major cellular sources of IFNγ	CD8+ and CD4+ T cells, NK cells
Effects of IFNγ	Regulates nearly all phases of immune and inflammatory responses, including the activation, growth and differentiation of T cells, B cells, macrophages, NK cells and others such as endothelial cells and fibroblasts. It enhances MHC Class II and FcR expression on macrophages, intracellular killing and ADCC activity Has weak antiviral and antiproliferative activity and promotes those activities of IFNα/β
Cross-reactivity	There is **no** cross-species reactivity

Table 6.6 Characteristics of interleukin-4

Major cellular sources of IL-4	Activated T cells, mast cells and bone marrow stromal cells
Effects of IL-4	IL-4 causes the activation, proliferation and differentiation of B cells. It is a growth factor for T and mast cells. It exerts other effects on granulocyte, megakaryocyte and erythrocyte precursors and macrophages. IL-4 induces IgG$_1$ and IgE secretion by murine B cells, and IgG$_4$ and IgE by human B cells
Receptors	Receptors are found on B and T cells, macrophages, mast cells and myeloid cells. Their number increases on cell activation
Cross-reactivity	There is **no** cross-species reactivity

Table 6.7 Characteristics of interleukin-5

Major cellular sources of IL-5	T cells, mast cells and eosinophils
Effects of IL-5	Stimulates eosinophil colony formation and eosinophil differentiation. Also acts as growth and differentiation factor for mouse (but **not** human) B cells
Cross-reactivity	There is considerable cross-species reactivity in functional assays

Table 6.8 Characteristics of interleukin-6

Major cellular sources of IL-6	B and T cells, monocytes/macrophages, bone marrow stromal cells, fibroblasts, keratinocytes, endothelial cells
Major inducers of IL-6	*Staphylococcus aureus* Cowan strain 1, IL-4, IL-1, TNFα, LPS, IL-6, IFNγ, PMA, GM-CSF, CSF-1, viruses, adherence, C5a, TNF
Effects of IL-6	Nuclear factor (NF)-IL-6 binds to the IL-6 multi-response element in the genome and is responsible for the induction of IL-6 in response to IL-1 and TNF. NF-IL-6 binds to the regulatory region of IL-8, G-CSF, IL-1, immunoglobulin, and the acute-phase protein genes, indicating that it may interact with many genes involved in acute-phase, immune and inflammatory responses
Cross-reactivity	Human IL-6 acts on mouse cells but **not** vice versa

Table 6.9 Characteristics of interleukin-13

Major cellular sources of IL-13	Activated T cells
Effects of IL-13	Inhibits production of inflammatory cytokines by LPS-stimulated monocytes (IL-1β; IL-6; TNFα: IL-8). Human and mouse IL-13 induce CD23 on human B cells, promote B cell proliferation in combination with anti-Ig or CD40 antibodies, stimulate secretion of IgM, IgE and IgG$_4$. Prolongs survival of human monocytes and increases expression of HLA-D and CD23. Human and mouse IL-13 have no known activity on mouse B cells
Cross-reactivity	IL-13 exhibits considerable cross-species reactivity

IL-4 has an autocrine effect on Th2 cells, specifically promoting their differentiation and proliferation. Characteristically, this results in the production of IgG$_4$ and IgE by human B cells.

Other cytokines are produced by both Th1 and Th2 cells, but are produced in far greater quantities by Th1 cells. These include granulocyte-macrophage colony-stimulating factor (GM-CSF; Table 6.10) and tumour necrosis factor (TNF).

An additional subset of Th cells has been described in mice — **Th0** — which has a pattern of cytokine secretion which is intermediate between those described for Th1 and Th2 cells. It is thought that these are **virgin cells**, i.e. those which have not encountered antigen. After stimulation, these cells may develop

Table 6.10   Characteristics of granulocyte-macrophage colony-stimulating factor

Molecular mass	Granulocyte-macrophage colony-stimulating factor (GM-CSF) has a molecular mass of 16.3 kDa (human), 16 kDa (murine). The molecule has two potential glycosylation sites and four cysteine residues. Disulphide bonding is important for biological activity of the molecule
Major cellular sources of GM-CSF	It is produced by activated lymphocytes, monocytes/macrophages, fibroblasts and endothelial cells
Effects of GM-CSF	GM-CSF promotes the growth and survival of haematopoietic progenitor cells; it stimulates formation of granulocytes, macrophages, mixed granulocyte–macrophage colonies and, at higher concentrations, eosinophil colonies from pluripotent stem cells. GM-CSF is bound by neutrophils, eosinophils and monocytes
Cross-reactivity	GM-CSF shows 56% homology in humans and mice; there is **no** cross-species activity

into Th1 or Th2 memory cells, which on subsequent exposure to antigen respond more rapidly, producing cytokines which will stimulate an appropriate response (either cell-mediated or humoral) to ensure the rapid elimination of the stimulating antigen.

The ability of memory T cells (both CD4+ and CD8+) to respond more quickly and strongly to antigen stimulation does not appear to be due to the expression of TCRs with increased affinity for antigen (i.e. T cells do not appear to exhibit affinity maturation) but rather to the altered expression of adhesion molecules such as CD2, LFA-1, LFA-3 and CD44 (ensuring enhanced interaction with antigen-presenting cells) and expression of IL-2 receptors which allow more rapid response to secreted IL-2 after activation.

Regulation of Th1 and Th2 Responses

IL-2 is the chief growth-promoting factor for both Th1 and Th2 subsets. In addition, IL-4 stimulates growth for a short time after encountering antigen. At later stages, Th2 cells still respond to both cytokines, whilst Th1 cells only respond to IL-2. As with naive cells, IL-1 is required as a co-stimulant after antigen presentation but only by Th2 cells. As mentioned earlier, IFNγ can inhibit the growth of Th2 cells by negating the effects of IL-4. In addition, Th2-produced cytokines are able to inhibit the production of IFNγ by Th1 cells and to suppress their growth. Thus, it appears that the outcome of a response to

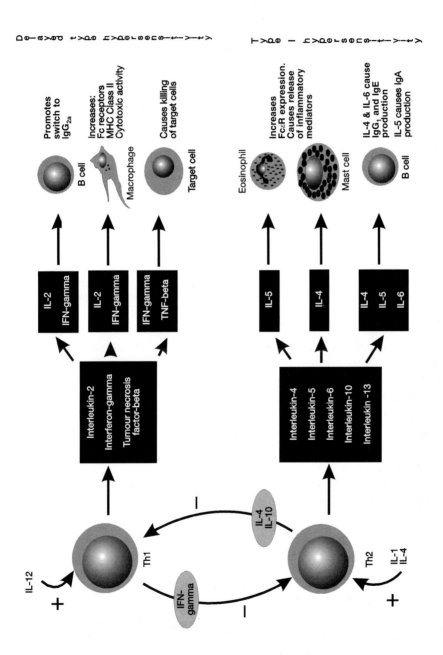

Figure 6.6 Regulation and outcome of Th1 and Th2 responses.

The outcome of a response to antigen depends on the balance of cytokines secreted. Initial responses may stimulate a Th1-type response, but if the antigen is not cleared, a Th2 response may develop

antigen depends on the balance of cytokines secreted (Figure 6.6). Initial responses may stimulate a Th1-type response, but if the antigen is not cleared, a Th2 response may develop. Such a change is observed in chronic *Mycobacterium tuberculosis* infections.

B CELL ADAPTIVE IMMUNITY

The B cell response to an antigenic challenge results in the production of specific antibody. The type of antibody and the kinetics of its production depend very much on whether or not it is the first time that the host has seen the antigen. In a secondary response, not only is the response much more rapid and of much greater magnitude, but also the antibodies show much higher affinity to the eliciting antigen. This change in antibody class and affinity is due to B cell maturation, differentiation and activation.

Upon first exposure to an antigen, a lag phase occurs, after which antibody of the IgM class which specifically recognises the eliciting antigen is produced. As the response continues, antigen-specific IgG is produced. This occurs much later in the response, reaches a plateau and then declines. Upon subsequent exposure to the antigen, a small IgM response occurs but a much larger IgG response develops very rapidly. Production continues to increase until a plateau is reached. This is at a much higher level than that observed in the primary response and declines very slowly, returning to base levels over a period of months or even years, depending on the eliciting antigen.

B Cell Differentiation and Antibody Production

Production of antigen-specific antibody by a B cell is the ultimate outcome of a complex, multistage differentiation. As mentioned in Chapter 1, B cells develop from **stem cells** in the bone marrow and are released into the bloodstream as mature cells which express antibody on their cell membrane (**mIg + B cells**). At a genetic level, this maturation can be explained by the rearrangement and expression of immunoglobulin heavy and light chain genes (Chapter 4). As the immune response to a T-dependent antigen matures, the predominating class of antibody changes from IgM to IgG, IgA or IgE. This may be explained by the **genetic switch hypothesis**, which proposes that in the primary repertoire, a given V region gene is brought into apposition with the μ chain gene. After interaction with an antigen, this same V region gene is rearranged next to another heavy chain gene, leading to a switch in the predominating antibody class which is seen during the maturation of an immune response. The expression of the $C\gamma$, $C\alpha$ or $C\varepsilon$ gene is accompanied by the simultaneous repression of the $C\mu$ gene.

Studies of serum antibody in a patient with multiple myeloma showed that the μ and γ chains had identical V region amino acid sequences. Since previous genetic studies had shown that constant domains of different heavy chains are synthesised by distinct structural genes, the myeloma protein studies suggested that heavy chain variable and constant regions are synthesised by different structural genes also. Thus, these experiments demonstrated that the different classes of antibody elicited by the same epitope had identical antigenic specificities and led to the determination that antibodies are the product of more than one gene.

B cell activation is regulated by the binding of lymphokines to their receptors and the interaction of cellular adhesion receptors. Once one set of signals has been received, the B cells express new or additional receptors which allow the cells to migrate to distinct microenvironments where they receive additional signals. Within the secondary lymphoid tissues (e.g. spleen and lymph nodes), most B cells are organised in the primary follicles of B-dependent areas. These areas also harbour some T cells and follicular dendritic cells (FDCs). After antigenic stimulation, germinal centres develop in these areas.

Some B cells are present in T areas where most of the T cells are organised in association with interdigitating cells (IDCs). In addition, some B cells are present in the marginal zones of spleen, where lymphocytes enter from the bloodstream and which contain marginal zone macrophages and a subset of dendritic cells. Thus, within each area, lymphocytes can be associated with different populations of accessory cells (IDCs, FDCs or macrophages) which are thought to play different roles during the various stages of B cell responses.

Primary response (virgin) B cells are highly T cell-dependent, their activation being MHC Class II restricted and requiring direct contact with T cells and the cytokines they produce. By contrast, secondary (memory) B cells require fewer T cells and less antigen. This probably reflects the requirement for antigen-presenting cells (such as macrophages and dendritic cells) to process and present antigen to virgin T cells. Once antigen-specific B cells exist, they bind antigen via their surface (Ig) receptors, process it and present it to memory T cells which produce the cytokines required for B cell activation. Antigen uptake via the B cell antigen receptor occurs at much lower levels of antigen than by endocytosis (Figure 6.7).

The change from a primary to a secondary immune response is characterised not only by an alteration in the predominant antibody class, but also by antibody maturation. This is the result of a series of complex, highly regulated events which results in the transition from the production of low-affinity

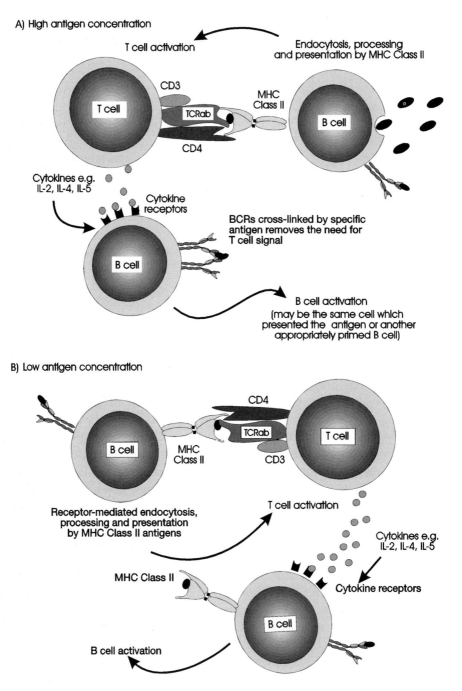

Figure 6.7   Antigen presentation by B cells.

Antigen-specific B cells bind antigen via their surface (Ig) receptors, and process and present the antigen to memory T cells which produce the cytokines required for B cell activation. Antigen uptake via the B cell antigen receptor occurs at much lower levels of antigen than by endocytosis

antibodies in the early primary response to high-affinity antibodies in the memory response. This maturation is dependent upon the occurrence of mutations in the heavy and light chain variable regions, the positive selection of advantageous mutants (which are given a considerable proliferative advantage over other cells) and the negative selection of those cells which have lost their capacity to recognise antigen. These selection processes, which are essential for the rapid development of the secondary response, depend on the ability of follicular dendritic cells within the germinal centres of the secondary lymphoid tissues to retain antibody–antigen complexes on their surface for long periods of time. Only activated B cells interact with these cells (since they do not express MHC Class II antigens), leading to their accumulation, differentiation and affinity maturation within the germinal centres.

Class Switching

Initially, B cells express mIgM and mIgD and, on any given cell, the variable regions of both IgM and IgD are identical, representing the association of different heavy chain constant region genes with a single variable region gene. Upon activation, these cells secrete IgM, the predominant antibody in a primary response. On secondary exposure to the antigen, other immunoglobulin classes predominate, i.e. IgG subclasses, IgE or IgA, representing the association of the original variable region gene with different heavy chain constant region genes. This **class switching** allows a cell to produce a different class of immunoglobulin (with different biological properties) whilst retaining the same specificity for antigen. It has been demonstrated in recent years that class switching is regulated by T cells and their soluble products, lymphokines. IL-4 has been shown to cause the switch to IgG_4 and IgE in humans (IgG_1 and IgE in mice). However, the switching process requires the presence of monocytes and physical interactions with T cells, since isolated B cells and purified IL-4 do not show class switching. The physical contact with T cells is thought to require the de novo expression of a surface antigen on activated cells which is the ligand for the CD40 molecule expressed on B cells. Indeed, antibodies to CD40 in association with IL-4 have been shown to negate the requirement for T cells in IgE switching.

The role of IFNγ in class switching has been clearly demonstrated in mice. This cytokine stimulates IgG_{2a} production in LPS-stimulated B cells. In addition, it stimulates the production of IgG_3 in B cells cultured with anti-Ig and IL-5. Despite this evidence in the murine model, there is no substantial evidence of a role for IFNγ in class switching in humans.

Finally, transforming growth factor-beta (TGFβ) has been shown to stimulate the switch to IgA production by pokeweed mitogen-stimulated human B cells. The switch also required T cell contact. However, the story cannot be that straightforward, since IgA production is mostly restricted to cells in mucosal-associated lymphoid tissue, whilst TGFβ is produced in numerous tissues.

LYMPHOCYTE MEMORY

Generally, the rapidity of secondary responses is a reflection, in part, of an increase in the number of antigen-specific precursor cells. However, this precursor frequency must be carefully regulated in order to limit the response to that required to eliminate a pathogen without causing incidental damage to the host. In order to understand how this regulation works, we must consider the cellular responses which occur during a primary immune response. Briefly, antigen localises in the lymphoid tissues (particularly in the paracortex of the lymph nodes and the periarteriolar lymphocyte sheaths of the spleen), where T and B cell primary responses are initiated. Naive lymphocytes recirculate through these areas and, upon recognition of antigen, the reactive cells are stimulated by lymphokines and rapidly proliferate in situ. The level of proliferation is dependent upon the concentration of antigen and the affinity of the receptors on the responding cells. Having acquired specific effector functions and the associated homing/adhesion molecules, the proliferating cells are released into the circulation. These new surface molecules allow the cells to attach to, and pass through, capillary walls, thus giving them access to tissues throughout the body. However, the primary response is usually short-lived, rapidly eliminating the stimulating antigen. The majority of the newly generated effector cells rapidly disappear, probably due to exhaustive differentiation and the effects of prolonged TCR signalling which may lead to the activation of intracellular pathways which induce a form of cell death known as apoptosis. Alternatively, effector cell death may be the result of a lack of growth-promoting lymphokines. This 'mass suicide' of effector cells may seem extravagant, but once the stimulating antigen is cleared, these cells are no longer required. Indeed, survival of these effectors could be deleterious, since the resulting response to antigen on second exposure would be excessive, leading to systemic shock. In addition, as more antigens were encountered, the increasing number of effector cells would eventually dilute out naive cells, reducing the ability of the host to mount a primary response to a new pathogen. However, it would also be wasteful if the immune system did not learn from its experience and so, in most instances, a proportion of the antigen-reactive cells become long-lived memory cells.

The development of T cell memory does not seem to reflect a random survival of effector cells since, with CD8 + cells at least, memory cells appear to have high-affinity receptors. Since T cells do not undergo somatic hypermutation, this affinity maturation may be the result of selective survival of high-affinity cells. By contrast, the development of B cell memory is characterised by **isotype switching** and **affinity maturation** caused by **somatic hypermutation**. This occurs in the germinal centres of secondary lymphoid tissues, an environment which appears to selectively promote the survival of high-affinity mutants. The survivors leave the germinal centres and become long-lived memory cells.

> Recent evidence from studies in mice suggests that virgin and memory cells may be derived from different precursor cells which are distinguished by different levels of expression of the heat-stable antigen (HSA) marker.

Memory T cells may be distinguished from naive cells by their surface antigen expression (Table 6.11) and by the cytokines they release after antigenic stimulation. In addition to the differential expression of those markers listed in Table 6.11, memory T cells express a range of surface antigens that are largely absent on naive cells. It has been shown that human T cells with a phenotype typical of memory cells divide much more rapidly than those with a naive T cell phenotype.

B cells also show phenotypic differences when they differentiate into memory cells. Naive cells generally express mIgM (in association with mIgD), whilst memory cells generally express mIgG, mIgA or mIgE. Additionally, memory B cells, like T cells, express higher levels of CD44 than naive B cells.

T and B memory cells are found throughout the secondary lymphoid tissues of the body. Experiments in animals have shown that lymphocytes (including memory cells) rapidly recirculate through both the blood and lymph. However, memory cells generally show decreased expression of L-selectin (the homing receptor for high endothelial venules in lymph nodes), suggesting that they may use a different recirculation pathway (such as via afferent lymphatic vessels) to naive cells. Since memory B cells tend to re-express L-selectin, only memory T cells may use this unusual route. It should be noted that not all memory cells recirculate.

Memory cells are thought to be resting and need to be reactivated to an effector state. However, memory T cells display many activation markers found on effector T cells. This has led to the suggestion that memory cells may be engaged in low-grade responses to persisting antigens and thus are **semi-activated**. Although memory is often long-lasting, it can decay quite rapidly (i.e. within several weeks), depending on the priming conditions.

Table 6.11 Characteristic expression of surface antigens on naive and memory T cells

	Naive T cells	Memory T cells
CD45R	High	Low
L-selectin	High	Low
CD44	Low	High

Evidence has shown that long-term memory cells are usually in G0 — the resting stage of the cell cycle. However, both T and B memory cells remain CD44 + for long periods; CD8 + cells have been shown to remain CD44 + for 18 months after adoptive transfer without specific antigen. This suggests that memory cells may not be resting but in a semi-activated state due to low-grade stimulation via T or B cell antigen receptors. This signalling is enough to maintain the expression of CD44 (and other activation markers) but not enough to cause the cells to enter the cell cycle. It has been suggested that the low-grade stimulation may be provided by cross-reacting environmental antigens.

Experiments in animals have suggested that the maintenance of memory depends upon the persistence of antigen. How can the priming antigen persist in the tissues for prolonged periods? Follicular dendritic cells are known to retain antigen on their surface for long periods. This antigen, if presented in association with MHC Class II products, can stimulate CD4 + cells. However, there is no evidence that these dendritic cells can present the same antigen in association with MHC Class I products to stimulate CD8 + cells. Thus, what is the explanation for CD8 + T cell memory? In the case of viral infections (which often elicit a CD8 + protective response), clearance of the organism in the primary response may be incomplete.

When primed B lymphocytes were adoptively transferred in mice in the absence of antigen, memory responses decayed rapidly. In contrast to this, co-transfer with antigen led to the maintenance of memory. Recently, similar dependence on antigen persistence has been demonstrated for both CD8 + and CD4 + T memory cells.

LEARNING OUTCOMES

Having completed this chapter you should have a good idea of how T cells and B cells are able to respond to antigenic stimulation on first and subsequent exposures. It is important to remember that the antigen receptor on T cells can only recognise antigen once it has been processed. In addition, it cannot recognise antigen alone; it must be presented to the T cells by products of the MHC. Any antigen-specific T cell response is dependent upon the activation of T helper cells which express CD4 molecules and must recognise antigen in association with MHC Class II gene products. These are expressed on professional antigen-presenting cells such as dendritic cells, macrophages and B cells. Once activated, T cells produce cytokines which stimulate B cells and other effector cells (such as cytotoxic T cells).

B cells (which do not need antigen to be presented to them and bind unprocessed antigen via mIg) proliferate and differentiate into plasma cells under the influence of T cell cytokines. Memory B cells have undergone an immunoglobulin class switch, which is also influenced by the cytokines produced by antigen-stimulated T cells.

Cytotoxic T cells are involved in the control of virus infections (these cells will be discussed in greater detail in Chapter 11). Most cytotoxic T cells (Tc) express the CD8 antigen. These cells recognise processed antigen which is presented by products of the MHC Class I genes. The latter are expressed by all nucleated cells, thus allowing the immune system to control potential virus infections in any cell of the body. Tc cells are activated by cytokines produced by Th cells.

Finally, you should have an understanding of how memory develops and the importance of this to the protection of the host from repeated exposure to infectious agents.

Chapter 7

Hypersensitivity

LEARNING OBJECTIVES

The purpose of this chapter is to introduce you to the term **hypersensitivity**, to explain what it means and to describe the immunological responses which accompany hypersensitivity reactions. When an antigen is introduced into an individual, the immune system recognises it as foreign and eliminates the invader in the most appropriate way, i.e. it limits any potential spread and destroys the antigen efficiently. The response is controlled such that only those mechanisms required are brought into play and there is little resulting tissue damage. However, in certain individuals the response to particular antigens may result in extensive tissue damage. It is accompanied by a massive **inflammatory response** which results in the signs and symptoms which are classified as hypersensitivity. Some people refer to this type of response as uncontrolled or harmful, but these are misnomers. It may be that in certain cases, e.g. in an infectious disease, the hypersensitivity response is vital to preventing the spread of the agent. Although tissue damage may result, the overall outcome is beneficial.

There are several different types of hypersensitivity reaction and we shall now consider them and the clinical conditions to which they give rise.

TERMINOLOGY

When an individual is exposed to an antigen, the outcome depends upon the strength of the immune response. At one extreme is **immunity** or **resistance** to the antigen and at the other is hypersensitivity, where the increased response to the antigen results in tissue damage. The scientist Paul Richet adopted the term **anaphylaxis** to describe the reaction which occurs in certain individuals to specific antigens. **Phylaxis** means 'protection', so anaphylaxis refers to the situation where damage occurs as a result of a protective response to a particular antigen. Thus, by these definitions, the terms hypersensitivity and anaphylaxis should be interchangeable. However, recently the use of the term anaphylaxis has been restricted to a very particular type of **hypersensitivity response**, the latter being a term used to describe any immunological reaction where considerable tissue damage occurs.

Another type of hypersensitivity response is the **allergic** response. The term **allergy** (from the Greek *allos* and *ergon* meaning 'altered action') was used initially to describe the outcome of the response to an antigen on second exposure.

HYPERSENSITIVITY REACTIONS

In recent years, research has shown that **hypersensitivity reactions** occur following re-exposure of an individual to an antigen to which he or she has previously been sensitised. This is similar to **immunisation**, where, on second exposure to an antigen, the host mounts a stronger, more efficient protective immune response than on initial exposure. The difference between this reaction and a hypersensitivity response is that the secondary response in the latter is so great that it causes varying degrees of tissue damage, resulting in the appearance of specific clinical signs and symptoms. Hypersensitivity can be caused by a wide range of antigens and may affect a number of different organs or tissues. In individuals where an antigen causes one particular type of hypersensitivity response — a type I response — the antigen is known as an **allergen** (i.e. **allergy generating**) and the clinical signs and symptoms characterise an allergic response. Allergies affect an increasing number of individuals every year (currently 20% of the population) and are an important cause of morbidity and mortality.

Hypersensitivity reactions were originally classified according to the symptoms which could be recognised in an individual. However, in the 1950s, Gell and Coombs proposed a classification system which depended upon the underlying immunological reactions. This system is used currently and the different types of hypersensitivity are discussed below.

Type I Hypersensitivity

Type I hypersensitivity reactions are becoming more common and you would recognise them as the signs and symptoms associated with allergic responses. Whilst the allergens (antigens) which stimulate these reactions are diverse, the outcomes of exposure to an allergen are similar. What determines whether or not an individual will respond normally to an antigen is not fully understood. Clearly there is a genetic influence, since family studies have shown that if both parents are allergic, an offspring has a 75% chance of being allergic. Only one parent being allergic reduces this to 50%. In addition, recent evidence suggests that the cellular interactions involved in antigen recognition and initiation of the immune response may influence the outcome.

Type I reactions are caused by the **inflammatory mediators** released from intracellular granules in basophils and mast cells as a result of cross-linking cell-bound IgE (Figure 7.1). Mast cells are found in connective tissues particularly around venules (CTMC), and in mucosal membranes (MMC). Although derived from the same progenitor cell under the influence of interleukin-3 (IL-3) (Table 7.1), the two types of mast cell show differences in the constitution of their cytoplasmic granules and their requirement for T cells, MMCs being unable to grow in the absence of T cells.

The large, cytoplasmic granules contain the chemicals which cause the signs and symptoms of **immediate hypersensitivity**, a massive inflammatory response. Some of these chemicals are listed in Table 7.2. Mast cells are triggered to degranulate by an allergen reacting with allergen-specific IgE bound to Fcε receptors (FcεR) on the mast cell surface. This interaction causes aggregation and reorientation of the receptors, resulting in degranulation of the mast cells.

The IgE receptor is made up of six chains, two α, two β and two disulphide-linked γ chains. One of the β and both of the γ chains are not exposed on the surface of the cells and are thought to be important in signal transduction and thus degranulation. The α chains comprise the binding site for the Fc portion of IgE. A lower-affinity FcεR (FcεRII) shows antigenic similarity to a B cell surface antigen — CD23 — which in soluble form may represent an IgE binding factor.

Type I reactions are also known as immediate hypersensitivity reactions, since they occur within seconds of exposure to the antigen. Examples of immediate hypersensitivity are shown in Table 7.3.

Regulation of Type I Hypersensitivity

Atopic diseases (allergies) are associated with elevated serum levels of both total and allergen-specific IgE. As mentioned above, immediate hypersensitivity results from the degranulation of mast cells/basophils caused by the cross-linking of cell-bound, antigen-specific IgE. The factors which regulate the production of IgE in response to an antigenic stimulus will clearly determine the outcome of exposure to that antigen. Usually, the primary response (characterised by the production of antigen-specific IgM) is followed, on subsequent exposure, by a secondary response typically characterised by the production of antigen-specific IgG (or, at mucosal surfaces, IgA). In certain individuals, antigen-specific IgE is produced after secondary exposure. This switch to IgE production is regulated by T cells through direct contact with B cells and the secretion of certain cytokines. The latter also affect other cells such as eosinophils, basophils and mast cells, which, upon activation, produce cytokines (such as IL-4 and IL-5) which exacerbate the allergic response (Figure 7.2).

As with immunisation, allergic sensitisation is initiated through the interaction of T cells, antigen-presenting cells and processed allergen. This

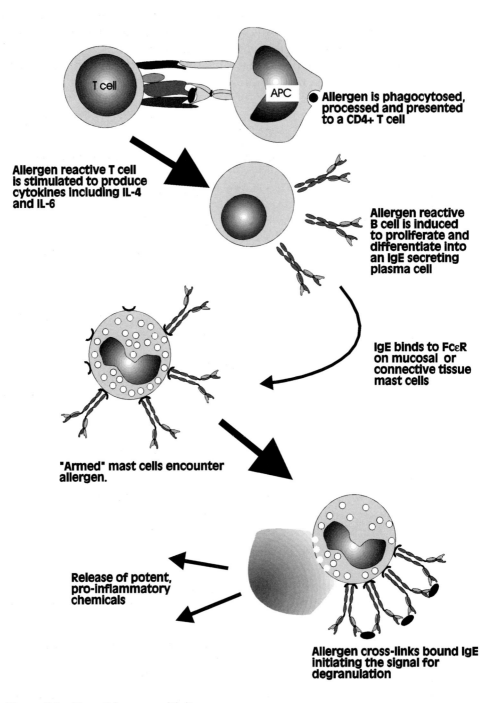

Allergen is phagocytosed, processed and presented to a CD4+ T cell

Allergen reactive T cell is stimulated to produce cytokines including IL-4 and IL-6

Allergen reactive B cell is induced to proliferate and differentiate into an IgE secreting plasma cell

IgE binds to FcεR on mucosal or connective tissue mast cells

"Armed" mast cells encounter allergen.

Release of potent, pro-inflammatory chemicals

Allergen cross-links bound IgE initiating the signal for degranulation

Figure 7.1   Type I hypersensitivity.

Type I reactions are caused by the inflammatory mediators released from intracellular granules in basophils and mast cells as a result of cross-linking cell-bound IgE

activation of naive T cells results in the production of cytokines such as IL-4 (produced by Th2 cells) or interferon-gamma (IFNγ) (produced by Th1 cells). It has been clearly demonstrated in animal models that stimulation of a Th2 response which leads to the production of IL-4 favours a B cell class switch

Table 7.1   Characteristics of interleukin-3

Characteristic	Description
Molecular mass	A haemopoietic growth factor of molecular mass 15.1 kDa (human), 15.7 kDa (mouse). The molecule has two potential glycosylation sites and one disulphide bond
Major cellular sources of IL-3	Produced by activated T cells, mast cells and eosinophils
Effects of IL-3	It supports the growth and differentiation of pluripotent stem cells, leading to the production of different blood cell types
Other names based on biological activity	Mast cell growth factor (MCGF); multi-colony-stimulating factor (M-CSF); eosinophil-CSF (E-CSF)
Genomic locality/organisation	Gene is on chromosome 5 in humans, and on chromosome 11 in mice
Cross-reactivity	Human and mouse IL-3 show only 29% homology. There is **no** cross-species reactivity

Table 7.2   Some pharmacological mediators in mast cell granules

Chemical	Effect
Histamine	Increases vascular permeability and levels of cAMP
Heparin	Causes anticoagulation
Serotonin	Increases vascular permeability
Chymase	Proteolysis
Hyaluronidase	Increases vascular permeability
Eosinophil chemotactic factor	Attracts eosinophils
Neutrophil chemotactic factor	Attracts neutrophils

Table 7.3   Examples of immediate hypersensitivity, their causes and outcome

Examples	Causes	Outcomes
Allergic rhinitis (hay fever) Bronchial asthma Atopic dermatitis	Varies between individuals, e.g.: ragweed or grass pollen, house dust mites	Symptoms result from antibody-bearing mast cells releasing histamine and other vasoactive amines

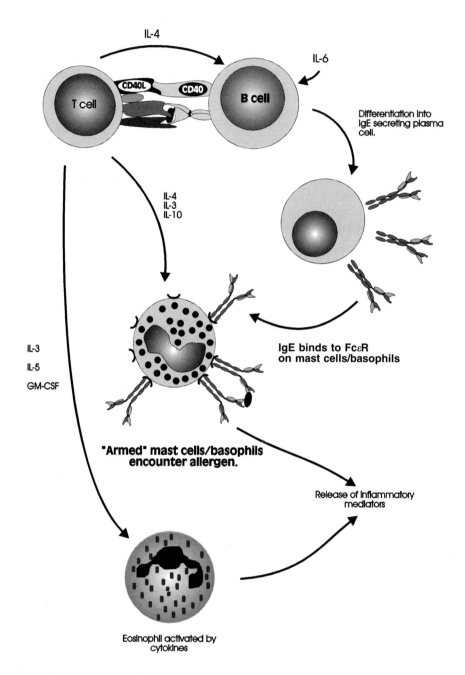

Figure 7.2 Cellular and molecular interactions leading to an allergic response.

In certain individuals, antigen-specific IgE is produced after secondary exposure to an antigen. This switch to IgE production is regulated by T cells through direct contact with B cells and the secretion of certain cytokines. The latter also affect other cells such as eosinophils, basophils and mast cells, which, upon activation, produce cytokines (such as IL-4 and IL-5) which exacerbate the allergic response from IgM to IgE production. IFNγ (from Th1 cells) inhibits IgE production as well as inhibiting the expansion of Th2 cells. So what makes an IgG response change to an IgE response? Experimental studies have suggested that antigens may deliver signals (via the TCR) that favour differentiation into Th2 cells. Complexes which bind the T cell receptor (TCR) with high avidity appear to favour the development of Th1-type responses. By contrast, weakly avid interactions favour the development of Th2-type responses. Cell surface molecules on both the T and antigen-presenting cells may influence the outcome of the TCR–MHC–allergen interaction. These molecules strengthen the contact between the cells or provide vital co-stimulatory signals.

The precise way in which the T cell–antigen-presenting cell–allergen interaction determines the type of Th response which follows is unknown but may be dependent upon differences in the signals transduced by interaction between the TCR–MHC and co-stimulatory molecules and their ligands leading to the transcription of different cytokine genes.

In addition to the subpopulations of Th (CD4+) cells, it has been suggested that CD8+ cells show similar subpopulations. Indeed, it has been shown that patients with allergies have a large subgroup of CD8+ T cells which produce IL-4 and stimulate IgE production in autologous B cells. As with Th cells, the development of type I and type II CD8+ subpopulations appears to be regulated by IFNγ and IL-4 respectively.

In addition to its release by T cells, IL-4 (and other cytokines such as IL-5) is produced by basophils, mast cells and eosinophils. These cytokines are vital to the differentiation, maturation and survival of effector cells (as shown for IL-5 and eosinophils). Thus, these cells modulate their own activity and perpetuate their participation in the allergic response. In addition, IL-4 provides a link between these effector cells and T cells, which is vital for the development of a Th2 response.

Type II Hypersensitivity

Under certain circumstances, an antibody (usually IgG or IgM) may recognise and bind to a normal or an altered cell surface antigen (Figure 7.3). Thus, the cell becomes part of an **immune complex** allowing activation of **complement** (via the classical pathway). This leads to the formation of the anaphylatoxins C3a and C5a which directly stimulate mast cells to degranulate, leading to an inflammatory response. Alternatively, the cell may become the target of an **antibody-dependent cellular cytotoxicity (ADCC)** reaction. These reactions result in tissue damage. Examples of this type of hypersensitivity include **erythroblastosis fetalis**, **myasthenia gravis** (a disease characterised by the presence of antibodies to the acetylcholine receptor) and **autoimmune haemolytic anaemia**.

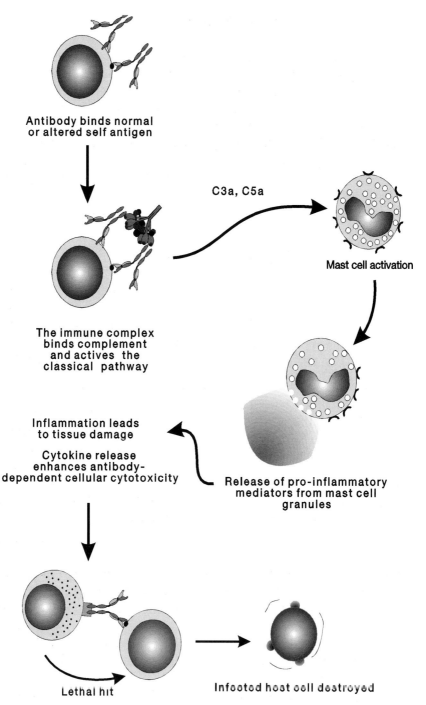

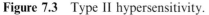

Figure 7.3 Type II hypersensitivity.

Under certain circumstances, an antibody (usually IgG or IgM) may recognise and bind to a normal or an altered cell surface antigen. This may lead to complement activation and the release of inflammatory mediators, resulting in tissue destruction

Type III Hypersensitivity

Type III hypersensitivity reactions are also the result of immune complex formation. Soluble antigen binds to specific antibody and may form large antigen–antibody lattices which can activate complement (Figure 7.4). These complexes can also be deposited in organs, particularly those with filtering membranes such as the kidneys and the joints. This type of hypersensitivity is responsible for the damage caused by inflammation in the glomeruli of the kidneys (**glomerulonephritis**) in a disease called **systemic lupus erythematosus** caused by DNA anti-DNA immune complexes. The distinction between type II and type III hypersensitivity is that the immune complexes which initiate the inflammation in the former contain cell-associated antigens.

Type IV Hypersensitivity

The final type of hypersensitivity is dependent upon the production of lymphokines resulting from the interaction of T cells with each other or with cells such as macrophages and fibroblasts. These reactions take more than 24 hours to develop and thus are also known as **delayed-type hypersensitivity** responses. Characteristics of these reactions are summarised in Table 7.4.

In 1890, Robert Koch demonstrated that filtrates from cultures of *Mycobacterium tuberculosis* could stimulate an inflammatory response several hours after injection into animals infected with the organism but not in uninfected animals. This technique has been developed and skin testing using preparations from a range of organisms is commonplace in detecting infected individuals and in screening populations to determine the prevalence of infection in specific communities.

The classic delayed-type hypersensitivity reaction is seen in response to the **purified protein derivative** of tuberculin (PPD) from *Mycobacteria* spp. If PPD is injected intradermally into an individual who has been exposed to *Mycobacterium tuberculosis* previously, there is no immediate reaction. After about 10 hours, the site of injection becomes red (erythema) and swollen, the reaction reaching a maximum between 24 and 72 hours. These classic signs of inflammation take several days to subside.

Histologically, the site of such a reaction is infiltrated with T cells and large numbers of newly recruited macrophages (monocytes) and mature macrophages. These cells are seen typically clustered around post-capillary venules. Deposition of fibrin is clearly evident and may be responsible for the solidity of the lesion.

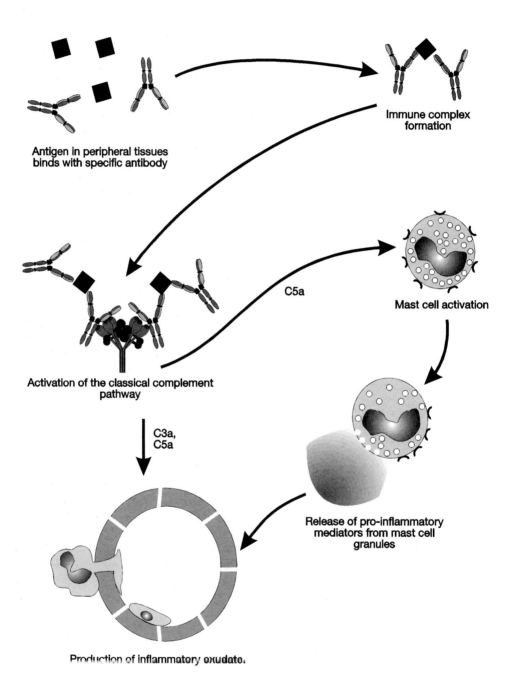

Figure 7.4 Type III hypersensitivity.

Soluble antigen binds to specific antibody and may form large antigen–antibody lattices which can activate complement. These complexes can also be deposited in organs, particularly those with filtering membranes such as the kidneys and the joints

Table 7.4 Summary of the characteristics of type IV hypersensitivity responses

Type	Onset	Duration	Characteristics
Contact	24 h	48–72 h	Macrophages; response occurs in the skin; thought to be due to Langerhans cells presenting antigen to CD4+ cells. CD8+ cells play a role, especially with haptens which modify MHC Class I antigens
Tuberculin type	24 h	72–96 h	Macrophages; antigen is presented by antigen-presenting cells such as dendritic cells and macrophages to CD4+ cells, which secrete cytokines, which recruit and activate macrophages. Th1 cells are particularly important in these reactions
Granuloma	7–14 days	Weeks	Macrophages and fibroblasts proliferate and produce collagen, which walls off the antigen. Giant cell formation occurs
Chronic basophilic hypersensitivity	12–24 h	24 h	Also called the Jones–Mote reaction. Only occurs in the epidermis. The principal cell type involved is the basophil but other granulocytes may be involved. The mechanism underlying the response is not well understood, and nor is its role. However, sensitivity is transferable with T cells, and it is thought that they secrete a lymphokine which is chemotactic for basophils

Immunologically, the basic mechanisms involved in a delayed-type hypersensitivity response are those seen in antigen-specific T cell responses. Antigen is taken up, processed and presented in association with MHC Class II molecules on the surface of dendritic cells, macrophages and possibly B cells. Antigen-specific CD4+ cells, typically Th1 cells, recognise the antigen and other co-stimulatory signals and secrete cytokines such as IFNγ and tumour necrosis factor, which stimulate changes in the local tissue macrophages, causing them to become activated. Once these cells are stimulated in this way, they release toxic substances (reactive oxygen and nitrogen intermediates) and cytokines which stimulate the inflammatory response and cause the destruction of both bacterial and tissue cells (Figure 7.5).

Activation of macrophages by IFNγ enhances the expression of MHC Class II antigens on these cells, providing a further stimulus for CD4+ cells, resulting in increased secretion of IFNγ. In addition, muramyl dipeptide (a component of mycobacterial cell walls) directly activates macrophages. Activation results in the production of a number of cytokines, but principally IL-1 and tumour necrosis factor. The former acts as a co-stimulator for T and B cells and, in synergy with IL-6, stimulates the secretion of IL-2 and the expression of IL-2

132

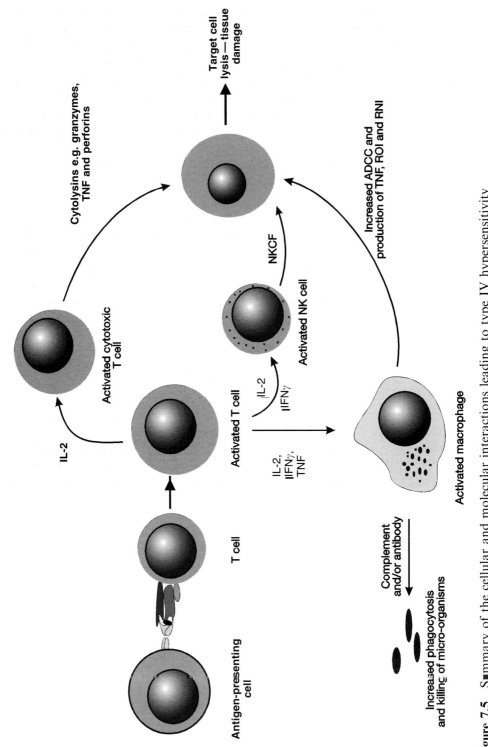

Figure 7.5 Summary of the cellular and molecular interactions leading to type IV hypersensitivity

receptors on T cells responding to antigenic stimulation. In addition, it is responsible directly or indirectly for many of the characteristics of inflammation; for example, it causes fever by stimulating the release of a pyrogen from the hypothalamus of the brain and synergises with tumour necrosis factor.

Tumour necrosis factor kills susceptible cells over a long period of time by mechanisms that are not wholly understood. Its cytolytic activity is increased by IFNγ and both act on neutrophils, increasing their phagocytic activity, superoxide anion production and antibody-dependent cellular cytotoxicity (ADCC).

In a delayed-type hypersensitivity reaction, direct activation of macrophages, e.g. by muramyl dipeptide in mycobacterial cell walls, in addition to the activation of T cells and the production of IFNγ and tumour necrosis factor, lead to the massive production of free radicals of oxygen and hydrogen peroxide, leading to extensive tissue damage. In many cases it is difficult to distinguish between a cell-mediated immune response and a delayed-type hypersensitivity response. Often, the only difference is the magnitude of the response and the degree of tissue damage which occurs, but it is a classic example of how hypersensitivity responses may be beneficial, since recovery from tuberculosis infection is always associated with tissue damage due to a delayed-type response.

LEARNING OUTCOMES

This chapter is designed to introduce the concept of hypersensitivity. After studying it, you should have a good understanding of the types of hypersensitivity responses which can occur, the mechanisms which underlie the resulting tissue damage and the stimuli for these responses. To find out if you have understood this chapter, test yourself using the associated program.

Chapter 8

Tolerance

LEARNING OBJECTIVES

In order for us to stay healthy, it is vital that our immune systems recognise and react to antigens derived from a variety of sources such as bacteria and viruses. You have already discovered how antigen must be processed and presented to T cells to stimulate an immune response. Antigen-presenting cells such as macrophages do not have the ability to specifically recognise an antigen; they present it regardless of its source. This could become problematic if these antigens are derived from our own cells (**self-antigens**). Generally, it is not beneficial for the immune system to recognise and react to self-antigens. Indeed, in most cases it is vital that the immune system tolerates 'self' and does not react to such antigens. But how can we explain this **tolerance**; the fact that an antigen normally found in our own body does not elicit an immune response whilst one which is not, does? Why do we live quite happily with our own organs, whilst one transplanted from someone else is rapidly rejected unless aggressive chemotherapy is employed? Originally, it was thought that all cells which showed reactivity to self-antigens were destroyed during development. However, there are a wide range of diseases in which the immune system does react to certain self-antigens. The existence of these **autoimmune diseases** suggests that the answer can not be that simple and that self-reactive cells must survive. The reactivity of lymphocyte clones is determined at a genetic level and thus it stands to reason that, due to certain events (such as random, somatic mutation), some self-reactive and therefore potentially damaging cells may develop.

Over the years, several areas of research have suggested the existence of a number of mechanisms by which **self-tolerance** is regulated. These mechanisms involve (1) the physical or functional neutralisation of self-reactive cells through **clonal deletion, clonal abortion** or **clonal anergy**, or (2) the control of autoreactive lymphocytes through the normal regulatory mechanisms of the immune system, e.g. through **idiotypic networks**. In this chapter you will see how self-tolerance is maintained by the mechanisms mentioned above. In addition, we shall look at the development of experimental tolerance. The factors regulating the ability to induce tolerance have many implications for our health. For example, antigens delivered in an appropriate manner will induce **immunity (immunisation)**, protecting the recipient against fatal infections; delivered in an inappropriate manner, the same antigen may induce tolerance, making the recipient highly susceptible to the infectious agent. Many other clinical applications for the development of tolerance exist (e.g. allergic desensitisation) and thus understanding the parameters which control tolerance is vital to such therapies.

LYMPHOCYTE TOLERANCE

As you have already discovered, products of the major histocompatibility complex (MHC) are found on the surface of all nucleated cells in the body. The structure of these molecules includes a cleft in which processed antigen is sited which may be presented to T cells (MHC Class I molecules to CD8+ cells and Class II to CD4+ cells). When processed foreign antigen is not available, peptides derived from the host's own proteins occupy these clefts. Since T cell antigen receptors are randomly generated, it is possible that a T cell would develop a receptor capable of recognising this processed self-peptide. If such development were uncontrolled, **self-reactive T cells** would be capable of initiating a response which would destroy those host tissues in which the original antigen was expressed. The situation is even more problematic with B cells. As you have seen, the generation of antibody diversity is a random process due to recombination and somatic mutation. B cells which recognise soluble, unprocessed antigen are capable (potentially) of generating antibodies which recognise any **antigenic epitope.** Antibodies recognising self-antigens could stimulate **complement activation** or **antibody-dependent cellular cytotoxicity (ADCC)**, leading to the destruction of the host's own tissues. Obviously, the capacity of T and B cells to react to self-antigens is clearly detrimental to the host, and a variety of mechanisms have developed to control or eliminate these self-reactive cells. This results in a state of non-responsiveness known as **immunological tolerance**. However, the efficiency of this process will depend on the mechanisms involved and the type of cell to be tolerised. The time required for the induction of tolerance, its duration and the level of antigen required to induce it will vary according to the type of cell involved, e.g. T or B lymphocyte.

Induction Time

Studies using cells from animals have given us an indication of the length of time required for the induction of tolerance in T and B cells (Table 8.1). However, it must be remembered that tolerance can be induced in vitro much quicker than in vivo and that induction times will vary somewhat between species and even between individuals.

Table 8.1   Time required for induction of tolerance in various cell types

Cell type	Antigen type	Time of induction
Splenic or thymic T cells		Within hours of challenge
Adult splenic B cells	T-dependent	Within 4 days of challenge
Mature bone marrow B cells	T-dependent	Within 15 days of challenge
B cells	T-independent	Quicker than T-dependent antigens due to higher avidity for B cell receptor

Lymphocytes are very susceptible to the induction of tolerance during fetal development and the first few weeks of life, i.e. before the immune system reaches maturity.

Thus, immature B cells are particularly susceptible whilst both mature B cells and plasma cells are relatively resistant. This difference in susceptibility is thought to be due to the modulation of antibody on B cells. Membrane immunoglobulin (mIg) is aggregated by antigen and is either endocytosed or shed from the cell surface. Until the mIg can be regenerated (or re-expressed), the cell is unable to respond to further antigenic stimuli, i.e. the individual is tolerant to the antigen. In mature B cells, the mIg is aggregated and removed from the cell surface in about an hour and is re-expressed after a few days. In addition, the process is rarely complete. By contrast, in immature B cells, this loss of mIg is more rapid and usually complete, and re-expression may take a very long time, if it occurs at all (Figure 8.1). Thus, tolerance is much easier to establish in immature B cells.

Antigen Dose

The level of antigen required to tolerise B cells is usually 100 to 1000 times greater than that needed for T cells (**high zone tolerance**). However, the required dose may be reduced if the B cell binds the tolerogen with high avidity. The dose of the antigen required will also vary according to the maturity of the cells. In contrast to mature B cells, neonatal B cells are much more susceptible to tolerance induction, and the level of antigen required to induce B cell tolerance in neonates is approximately 100-fold less than that required in adults. This is probably due to the lower concentration of mIg requiring cross-linking by antigen.

In addition to high zone tolerance, some weak immunogens may be given at very low levels and result in **low zone tolerance**. However, this form of tolerance has limitations, in that it is usually only partially effective, only affecting some cells, and is maintained by a subpopulation of T cells. These cells suppress the activity of the potentially autoreactive B cells. It is thought that the extremely low levels of antigen selectively activate these T suppressor cells; T helper cells require much higher doses of antigen in order to be activated.

Mature B cells

Immature B cells

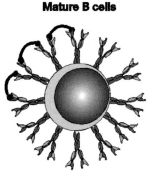

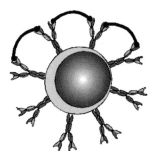

**Antigen aggregates mIg which
is endocytosed or shed after 1 hour**

**mIg is rapidly aggregated and
endocytosed or shed**

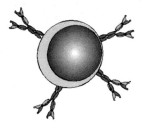

Only partial loss of receptors

Loss of mIg is usually complete

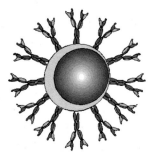

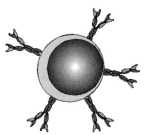

**Re-expression of mIg after
a few days**

**If re-expression of mIg occurs at all
it may take a very long time to be complete**

**SHORT-LIVED TOLERANCE
DIFFICULT TO INDUCE**

**LASTING TOLERANCE
EASILY INDUCED**

Figure 8.1   B cell tolerance.

In mature B cells, mIg may be aggregated by antigen and removed from the cell surface in about an hour and is re-expressed after a few days, although the process is rarely complete. By contrast, in immature B cells, this loss of mIg is more rapid and usually complete, and re-expression may take a very long time, if it occurs at all

Antigen Persistence

Generally, antigen must be continually present to maintain tolerance. Thus, tolerance which follows a single injection of an antigen which is only removed and digested slowly is more persistent than that induced by antigens which are rapidly cleared from the system.

Specificity

When tolerance is induced, the host fails to respond to a particular **antigenic determinant**. Thus, if the determinant is a common one which appears in a number of different antigens, the host will be tolerant to that antigenic determinant in all the antigens in which it is expressed. If the determinant is the **major immunogenic determinant** (i.e. it is the determinant which is primarily responsible for eliciting an immune response to those antigens), then the host will be tolerant to a range of antigens (Figure 8.2). If, however, the antigens express other immunogenic determinants, then the host will be able to respond to them and clear the antigen from the system.

Duration

It is difficult to envisage how, if a self-reactive cell has been deleted, self-reactivity can re-emerge. Self-reactivity is determined by the specificity of the T cell receptor (TCR) or B cell receptor (BCR). Since these receptors are generated by recombination events between several genes and by somatic mutation, the new cells being produced by the bone marrow may, by chance, develop further self-reactive receptors. Thus, when tolerance is due to clonal deletion, recovery is related to the time required to regenerate mature lymphocytes from the stem cell population. However, if tolerance is caused by blockade of antibody-forming cells, this is rapidly lost by removal of the antigen. In general, T cell tolerance is more persistent than B cell tolerance.

Route of Administration

We have already mentioned how the dose of an antigen may affect tolerance induction. In addition, the route of administration may influence which cells become tolerised to a particular dose. For example, a given dose of an antigen may induce tolerance in both B and T cells when given internally. However, when applied to the skin, the same dose may induce an antibody response but fail to stimulate a cell-mediated response. In such a situation, the T cells responsible for the stimulation of a delayed-type hypersensitivity response are

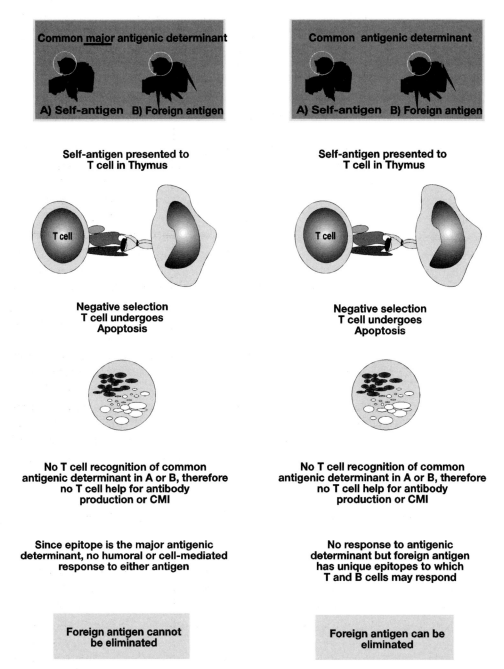

Figure 8.2   Effect of tolerance to a major immunogenic determinant.

When tolerance is induced, the host fails to respond to a particular antigenic determinant. Thus, if the determinant is a common one which appears in a number of different antigens, the host will be tolerant to that antigenic determinant in all the antigens. If the determinant is the major immunogenic determinant, then the host will be tolerant to a range of antigens tolerised whilst other T cells and B cells are not. This implies that not only do B and T cells show differences in susceptibility to tolerance induction, but that also subpopulations of T cells are differentially affected (in this case it is likely that Th1-type cells are tolerised whilst Th2-type cells are not).

Tissue Specificity

Some tissues in the body exhibit surface antigens which are peculiar to that tissue. In addition, the expression of certain antigens is associated with the stage of development or maturation of a particular cell. Although blood cells derive from the bone marrow, they may express antigens associated with their mature status that are not expressed on the immature precursors in the bone marrow. Thus, an animal (A) tolerised by the neonatal injection of bone marrow haemopoietic cells from another strain (B) may not be tolerant to an injection of blood from B. This is due to the host recognising foreign antigens on the strain B mature blood cells which are not expressed on the strain B haemopoietic cells to which it has become tolerant.

Since the majority of self-reactive T and B cells are eliminated in the primary lymphoid tissues (the thymus and bone marrow respectively), lymphocytes capable of recognising an antigen whose expression is limited to a tissue distinct from these will escape destruction. In the periphery, these potentially autoreactive cells must be controlled to prevent disease. If the antigen is expressed in an **immunologically privileged site** (i.e. immunological cells do not normally have access to it), e.g. the brain, the autoreactive cells are unlikely to cause disease unless tissue damage (e.g. due to virus infection) causes the release of the antigen or recruitment of immunologically active cells to the site.

MECHANISMS OF TOLERANCE INDUCTION

The interaction between an antigen and its specific cell surface receptor may result either in the activation and differentiation of the cell (**positive selection**) or in its inactivation or even death (**negative selection**). Positive selection usually results in a cell leaving G_0 and entering the cell cycle, giving rise to a clone of increasingly differentiated effector cells, e.g. cytotoxic T cells and plasma cells. This process is known as **clonal selection**. By contrast, when an antigen–receptor interaction results in negative selection leading to cell death, it is known as **clonal deletion** (Figure 8.3). Although only a single cell is destroyed, the host has lost the potential to develop the **clone** of cells which would recognise the epitope in question. When the self-reactive cell is not killed but made functionally inactive, the outcome is known as **clonal anergy**.

The theory of clonal deletion was first proposed by Burnett to explain the lack of self-reactivity in the immune system. This suggested that all cells bearing

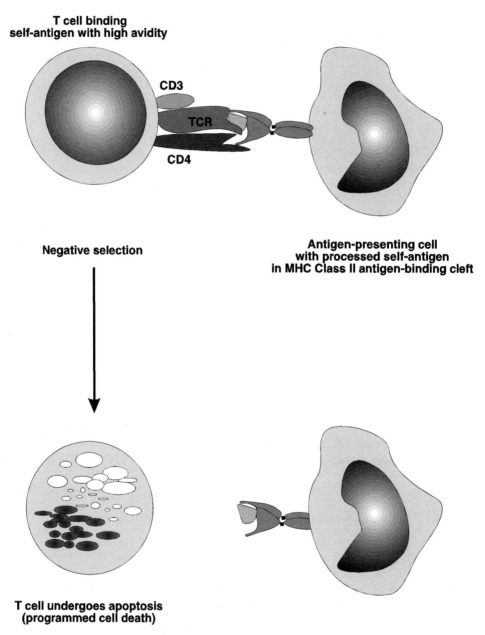

T cell binding self-antigen with high avidity

CD3

TCR

CD4

Negative selection

Antigen-presenting cell with processed self-antigen in MHC Class II antigen-binding cleft

T cell undergoes apoptosis (programmed cell death)

Figure 8.3   Clonal deletion. When an antigen–receptor interaction results in negative selection leading to cell death, it is known as clonal deletion

receptors which recognise self-antigen were destroyed, thus preventing the development of an **autoimmune response**. Death usually results from the induction of **apoptosis** (often referred to as cellular suicide or programmed cell death) in the self-reactive cells.

AUTOIMMUNE RESPONSE

This is directed against antigens expressed by the host's own tissues (auto) and leads to tissue damage. If the antigen is restricted to one particular organ or tissue (e.g. the thyroid), the resulting signs and symptoms are typical of a disease affecting that organ. However, if the antigen is expressed in several tissues or organs, the signs and symptoms will be more generalised.

Since immunological activation depends on the concentration of the antigen and the level of receptor expression, some self-reactive cells may not be activated by the local antigen concentration or may not express high enough levels of receptor molecules under normal circumstances. Such cells would not be subject to negative selection but also would not normally cause disease. However, should circumstances change, i.e. an increase in local antigen concentration due to tissue damage, the cell may be activated and autoimmune damage would result. This type of non-reactivity has been called **clonal ignorance**.

Mechanisms Inducing Tolerance in B Cells

B cell tolerance has been described as 'the absence of a measurable antibody response to an antigenic challenge'. In order that tolerance might be established, antigen must bind the BCR. However, in only a few cases does this interaction lead to tolerance rather than to activation and antibody formation. Several mechanisms have been proposed to explain the regulation of autoantibody production.

Clonal Abortion

If immature B cells developing in the primary lymphoid tissues (e.g. the bone marrow) are exposed to extremely low levels of specific antigen for the first time, normal maturation is inhibited and the cell is unable to respond appropriately upon subsequent challenge. This type of tolerance is known as **clonal abortion** and is easily induced.

Clonal Exhaustion

Repeated challenge with immunising doses of a T-independent antigen may cause **clonal exhaustion**. This type of antigen usually stimulates mIgM + cells and does not cause the formation of memory cells. The stimulated cells differentiate into antibody-producing cells which are only short-lived, and after each challenge, fewer cells remain which are capable of responding, until eventually all reactive cells are exhausted (Figure 8.4). When self-antigens are the stimulating agent, their continued presence ensures clonal exhaustion. With non-self-antigens, removal of the agent will allow clonal recovery over an extended period of time.

Clonal Deletion

Clonal deletion has been demonstrated (in mice) to be responsible for the elimination of B lymphocytes reactive with cell surface-bound self-antigen. Even antigens which have low affinity for the B cell antigen receptor can induce deletion. Depending on where the cells are exposed to autoantigen, deletion can occur in the pre-B to B cell transitional stage or after the cells leave the bone marrow.

Clonal Anergy

T-dependent antigens. The mechanisms controlling B cell tolerance to T-dependent antigens are difficult to define, since T helper cells may recognise determinants on the antigen, enabling them to trigger B cells. Thus, tolerance to these antigens can only be induced if the host lacks functional T cells or the T cells are effectively tolerant to determinants on the antigen.

The response of B cells to T-dependent antigens is dependent upon signals received from antigen-specific T cells. If this T cell help is not provided, the B cell cannot respond and is considered to be functionally deleted. This results in clonal anergy.

T-independent antigens.   B cells may be tolerised to a variety of T-independent antigens which, generally, are slowly metabolised in vivo and tend to promote relatively long-lasting tolerance. The degree of tolerance and its persistence is dependent on the dose of antigen injected.

To act as effective tolerogens, T-independent antigens are required in higher doses than T-dependent antigens.

T-independent antigens are usually large molecules made of repeating subunits and have a high number of identical antigenic determinants. Such molecules are capable of cross-linking a large number of antigen-specific receptors on B cells and in this way may eliminate the need for T cell help. If such a T-independent antigen is present at too high a concentration or is present in a non-immunogenic form, abnormal intracellular signals are produced which fail to trigger proliferation and differentiation of the B cells, i.e. they are functionally deleted or clonally anergic.

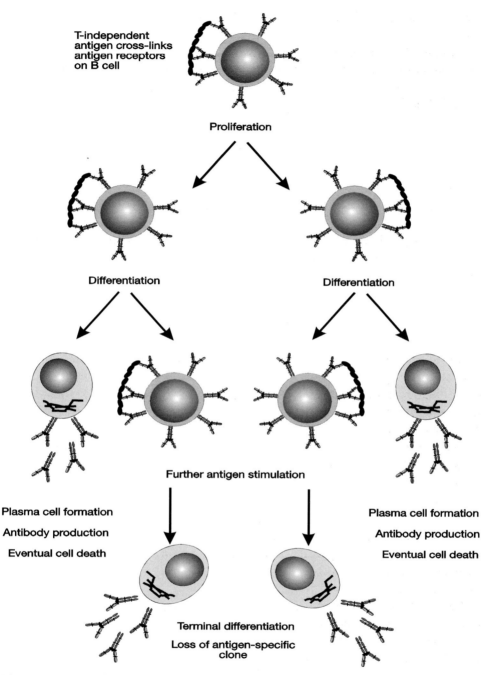

Figure 8.4 Clonal exhaustion.

Clonal exhaustion results from repeated challenge with immunising doses of a T-independent antigen (TI). TI antigens usually stimulate mIgM+ cells and do not stimulate memory cell production. Stimulated cells differentiate into short-lived antibody-producing cells, and after each challenge, fewer cells remain until eventually all reactive cells are exhausted

Antibody-forming Cell (AFC) Blockade

Although it is very difficult to tolerise antibody-forming cells, very large doses of T-independent antigens can sometimes be effective. The process is similar to that described above, in that high concentrations of antigen blockade the antigen receptors of the antibody-forming cell and, in doing so, interfere with antibody secretion.

Antibody-induced Tolerance

When the V region of an antibody is formed by somatic mutation and recombination events, the resulting protein is unique. Thus, the antigen-binding site, which is made up of the V regions of the heavy and light chains and is known as the **idiotype** of the antibody, may be considered to be foreign to the host — since the immune system has not been exposed to it previously. Thus, the antigen-binding site of an antibody may act as an antigen itself and induce the formation of specific antibody. As with any antigen, it may be made up of many antigenic determinants which (in this case) are known as **idiotopes**. Antibodies which recognise these idiotopes are called **anti-idiotypic antibodies**. Thus, anti-idiotypes are specific for the antigen-binding sites which induced their formation, and if these are part of the immunoglobulin molecules on the surface of a B cell, the anti-idiotypes will cause the mIg to be cross-linked. This may lead to tolerance if the appropriate concentration of anti-idiotype is present (Figure 8.5). The effect of such tolerance is to prevent the B cell from responding to its eliciting antigen. It is thought that this mechanism is involved in the 'switching off' of an immune response.

Mechanisms Inducing Tolerance in T Cells

The ways in which T cells are tolerised are similar in some ways to those in which B cells are tolerised. However, unlike B cells, T cells are functionally diverse and require quite complex cellular interactions to occur before they can recognise antigen.

The principal mechanisms involved in establishing T cell tolerance are clonal deletion in the thymus and clonal anergy in the periphery. However, these mechanisms are not completely effective, and self-reactive T cells are found in the circulation of normal individuals. However, these cells probably exhibit too weak an affinity for self-antigen to be eliminated in the thymus or to cause autoimmune disease under normal circumstances

Clonal deletion of autoreactive T cells in the thymus is clearly influenced by thymic epithelial cells. In addition, clonal anergy in the periphery is thought to be influenced by bone marrow-derived antigen-presenting cells which can induce tolerance rather than activation under certain circumstances.

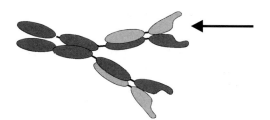

**The antigen-binding site
— the idiotope — is a unique
conformation of amino
acids and as such may be
immunogenic.**

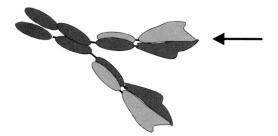

**An anti-idiotype is an antibody
whose production has been
stimulated by a particular
idiotype and whose antigen-
binding site is specific for the
idiotope of the eliciting antibody.**

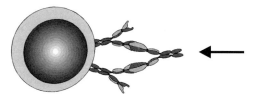

**Anti-idiotype antibody cross-
links idiotypes on B cell surface.
Resulting signal induces tolerance.**

Figure 8.5   Anti-idiotypic antibodies.

The antigen-binding site of an antibody is known as the idiotype; this may act as an antigen itself and induce the formation of specific antibody. As with any antigen, it may be made up of many antigenic determinants, which (in this case) are known as idiotopes. Antibodies which recognise these idiotopes are called anti-idiotypic antibodies. Thus, anti-idiotypes are specific for the antigen-binding sites which induced their formation, and if these are part of the immunoglobulin molecules on the surface of a B cell, the anti-idiotypes will cause the mIg to be cross-linked. This may lead to tolerance if the appropriate concentration of anti-idiotype is present

Clonal Deletion

Clonal deletion in the thymus is thought to play a role in the development of T cell tolerance. It has been demonstrated using foreign antigens in animals that it is easy to induce tolerance through clonal deletion in the embryo or in neonatal life, but not in the adult. This is thought to be due to mature T cells preventing the deposition of the antigen in the adult thymus.

T cells capable of recognising self-antigens are deleted in the thymus during their differentiation (Figure 8.3). Positive selection within the thymus ensures that all mature T cells are able to recognise the proteins coded for by the MHC on all cells of the body. On the other hand, negative selection ensures that most potentially damaging self-reactive T cells are identified and effectively neutralised by ensuring that they come in contact with a mixture of self-antigens within the thymic environment. The elimination of self-reactive T cells is thought to be dependent upon the avidity with which the T cell binds the antigen. T cells expressing receptors which bind antigens with only low affinity may escape elimination and pass into the periphery.

Maintenance of T Cell Tolerance

A number of processes have been identified which regulate T cell tolerance. The initial step occurs in the thymus and is clonal deletion of T cells with receptors which recognise self-antigen with high affinity. However, due to their recognition of short linear arrays of amino acids, T cells have a limited repertoire (when compared to B cells) and so the threshold of clonal deletion must be set low enough to ensure that a wide repertoire of T cells is available in the periphery to combat foreign antigens. This means that T cells whose antigen receptors have an affinity for self-antigens below the threshold avoid clonal deletion, mature and enter the circulation. In addition, T cells which recognise antigenic epitopes derived from self-peptides which are not expressed or presented in the thymus will also escape.

Those cells which are not deleted in the thymus but which show some measure of self-recognition may be controlled by other tolerance-inducing mechanisms. These include altered signal transduction (resulting in clonal anergy) and alteration of the expression of co-receptor and accessory molecules, resulting in reduced affinity of the antigen receptor. In addition, suppression of T-cell responses has been clearly observed but the precise mechanisms involved are unclear.

Mechanisms Involved in the Development
of Incomplete Tolerance

Tolerance induction may involve the deletion of only some aspects of the immune response, which results in incomplete tolerance. For example, if T cell tolerance is induced to an antigen, B cells may still be able to respond. If the T cells are only tolerant to a single antigenic determinant on the antigen, help for B cells may be provided by T cells reacting to other determinants on the antigen (Figure 8.6).

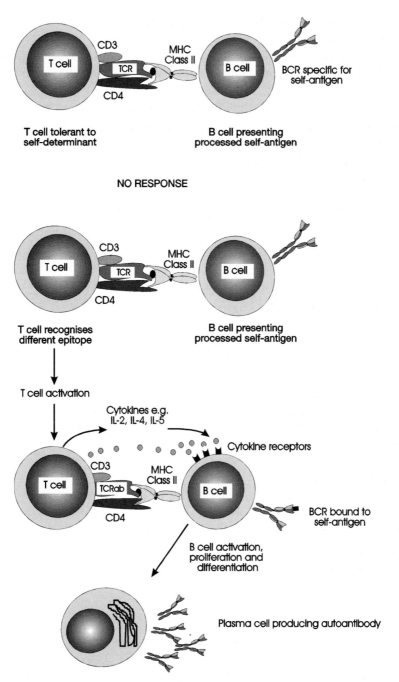

Figure 8.6 Induction of partial tolerance.

Tolerance induction may involve the deletion of only some aspects of the immune response, which results in incomplete tolerance. If T cells are only tolerant to a single antigenic determinant on an antigen, help for B cells may be provided by T cells reacting to other determinants on the antigen

Affinity and Isotype Maturation

A secondary antigen-specific antibody response involves a switch from IgM to IgG production and an increase in antibody affinity. However, after tolerisation, the antibody response may fail to mature in the normal way, and a secondary antigenic challenge may result in an abnormal spectrum of antibody classes or antibodies of lower affinity than expected. This may be due to the preferential tolerisation of high-affinity B cells, blockade of antibody-forming cells of a particular isotype and/or the selective action of T cell subpopulations resulting in suppression.

B cells show differences in sensitivity to tolerance induction, depending on their mIg class. Thus, T-independent antigens induce tolerance in B cells in the following order: mIgE + > mIgG + > mIgM +; some T-dependent antigens show preferential induction in $mIgG_2$ + cells rather than $mIgG_1$ + cells.

LEARNING OUTCOMES

Having read this chapter, you should have a good appreciation of the mechanisms which control the outcome of exposure to an antigen. During fetal development, nascent T and B cells are exposed to a wide variety of self-antigens and are selected for survival or death based on the avidity with which they bind these antigens. However, it is not possible for all antigens to be presented to these developing cells — some antigens are only present in one type of tissue which may not normally be exposed to the immune system. Thus, T or B cells capable of recognising such antigens will not be deleted in the primary lymphoid tissue but must be regulated in the periphery to prevent the development of autoimmune disease.

A number of factors affect the ease with which tolerance may be induced, and subpopulations of cells show different levels of susceptibility. You should now read some of the recommended texts to see how an understanding of the mechanisms controlling tolerance can influence the approaches taken to develop vaccines. Breakdown of tolerance leads to the development of autoimmune disease, which we will discuss in the next chapter.

Chapter 9

Autoimmune Diseases

LEARNING OBJECTIVES

The purpose of this chapter is to introduce you to the concepts of **autoimmunity** and **autoimmune disease** and to distinguish between them. A number of familiar diseases may be considered to be autoimmune in nature, e.g. **rheumatoid arthritis** and **multiple sclerosis**. This means that the majority of the tissue damage observed in these diseases (**pathology**) occurs as a result of the immune system failing to maintain tolerance to self. Usually in autoimmune diseases, the **immunopathology** may be the result of one or more hypersensitivity reactions. We shall now consider all these aspects of autoimmunity in more detail, giving examples of autoimmune diseases to illustrate the points made.

AUTOIMMUNITY

Autoimmunity, as opposed to autoimmune disease, is vital to the development of a normal immune response. As we discussed in Chapter 5, T cells recognise antigen only in association with self-MHC molecules; they will not respond if the antigen is presented by foreign MHC molecules, thus confirming that the reaction involves specific recognition of self molecules. This is an example of autoimmunity which is productive. A further example is the recognition of self-idiotypes by anti-idiotypic antibodies, which is essential for the diversification and regulation of immune responses. Apart from these instances, the immune system does not normally react to itself, i.e. it is **tolerant to self**.

Self-tolerance occurs early in fetal development and is vital for health and the normal functioning of the immune response; its breakdown results in autoimmune disease, which may be debilitating or even fatal. How can such autoimmunity develop? One suggestion is that an antigen may be hidden from the immune system during development (e.g. an antigen within an organ which has little contact with immunologically active cells — an immunologically privileged site), thus preventing the development of tolerance to that antigen at the T or B cell level. If the antigen is exposed later in life as a result of some form of tissue damage, it will be foreign to the immune system and it will stimulate an (auto)immune response. This type of response may be a primary cause of, or a secondary complication in, a variety of human and animal diseases.

Many studies have demonstrated that self-reactive lymphocytes are part of the normal immunological repertoire and only a small fraction of these cells may be pathogenic, the remainder having a physiological role to play.

Causes of Autoimmunity

Every day, the body is exposed to a number of factors which alone, or in combination, under the correct conditions may initiate the development of an autoimmune disease. In addition, it is also a normal consequence of ageing and may be induced by certain drugs or micro-organisms (especially viruses). The exact cause of most autoimmune diseases is largely unknown, as are the factors which control the severity of the disease, the range of autoantigens or the target organs involved. However, a number of parameters are known to be generally associated with autoimmune disease and these are discussed briefly in the following sections (Table 9.1).

Genetic Factors in Autoimmune Disease

The genetic make-up of the host may be a major determinant in the onset and development of autoimmune disease. Particularly relevant in this respect are those genes which control the size and type of immune response to an antigen, i.e. the MHC and antigen receptor genes. Several autoimmune diseases have been shown to be associated (at least loosely) with the expression of particular MHC and immunoglobulin allotypic genes. Individuals with **seropositive rheumatoid arthritis (RA +)** commonly express the product of the Class II gene DR4, whilst **systemic lupus erythematosus (SLE)** is associated with DR2 and DR3. Although these diseases are commonly thought to be closely related, the distinct genetic association suggests that their pathology may be very different.

Modern developments in molecular biology have provided the potential for developing new types of treatment for autoimmune diseases, such as gene therapy. However, further progress is required before it becomes the treatment of choice. First, the genes involved in each disease must be isolated and characterised, and delivery systems allowing efficient gene insertion in the target cells must be developed, as must the mechanisms to regulate expression of the introduced genes.

Sex-linked Factors in Autoimmune Disease

Generally, women are much more susceptible than men to most connective tissue diseases which include autoimmune diseases. The incidence of the latter is

Table 9.1   Factors affecting the development of autoimmune disease

Agent	Effects/Associated autoimmune disease
Genetic make-up	HLA-DR4 — rheumatoid arthritis HLA-DR2, 3 — systemic lupus erythematosus HLA-DQ3 — insulin-dependent diabetes mellitus
Viruses	e.g. Epstein–Barr virus
Hormones	Oestrogen aggravates autoimmune disease; androgens are immunosuppressive
Stress/Trauma	Neurochemicals and hormones are involved in rapid onset of autoimmune disease in response to these agents
Pharmaceuticals	
Lithium	Autoimmune thyroid disease
Penicillin	Autoimmune haemolytic disease
Penicillamine	Myasthenia gravis, pemphigus, autoimmune thyroid disease, autoimmune haemolytic anaemia
α-Methyldopa	Autoimmune haemolytic anaemia, autoimmune hepatitis
Chemicals and organic solvents	
Hydrazine	Systemic lupus erythematosus
Vinyl chloride, silica dust	Systemic sclerosis
Heavy metals	
Gold, cadmium, mercury	Immune complex glomerulonephritis
Food additives	
Tartrazine	Systemic lupus erythematosus

demonstrably affected by both sex hormones and genes linked to the X or Y chromosomes. It is well known that many hormones affect the lymphoid system; the effect of gonadal hormones is particularly apparent. Indeed, it has been shown that elevated oestrogen levels exacerbate autoimmune disease whilst androgen has a protective, immunosuppressive role.

Stress and Neurochemicals in Autoimmune Disease

Many instances are cited in the clinical literature where patients have had a dramatic onset of autoimmune disease following trauma or extreme stress. Neurochemicals and hormones are thought to play a vital role in initiating disease under these circumstances.

Chemicals and Pharmaceuticals in Autoimmune Disease

With the worldwide explosion of manufacturing industry and pollution, an association between exposure to certain chemicals and the development of specific autoimmune diseases has been clearly established. These agents may interact with tissues, resulting in the expression of modified self-antigens which are the target for an autoimmune response. Similarly, pharmaceuticals may induce disease. For example, treatment with methyldopa has been associated with the development of **autoimmune haemolytic anaemia**.

Viruses in Autoimmune Disease

Viruses have been found to be associated with the presence of autoimmune disease in humans and other animals. They may cause autoimmune disease by a number of different mechanisms, including polyclonal activation of lymphocytes (e.g. Epstein–Barr virus), release of intracellular organelles due to destruction of host cells, antigen mimicry (Figure 9.1; Table 9.2), induction of abnormal MHC Class II antigen expression and functional impairment of immunologically regulatory cells, e.g. T suppressor cells.

Role of Epstein–Barr virus in autoimmune disease.   Epstein–Barr virus (EBV) infects B cells and directly causes their activation. Although some autoreactive B cells escape elimination in the bone marrow, they are usually prevented from producing autoreactive antibody either by a lack of antigen-stimulated T cell help or by T cell-mediated suppression. However, if a potentially autoreactive B cell is infected by EBV, it can proliferate and differentiate into a plasma cell without the help of T cells. Infected cells from both healthy individuals and patients with rheumatoid arthritis secrete polyclonal IgG and IgM anti-immunoglobulin antibodies (rheumatoid factor) but B cells from patients produce more, higher-affinity antibody than those from normal persons.

CLASSIFICATION OF AUTOIMMUNE DISEASE

In the 1950s, Witebsky established the criteria for determining the aetiology of human diseases which were thought to be autoimmune. Witebsky's postulates were modelled on those of Koch and required the presence of autoantibody or a cell-mediated immune response to a self-antigen which had been identified as inducing a similar disease in an experimental host mediated by the same immunological mechanism. Since these criteria were established, our knowledge of immunology has increased by leaps and bounds. However, they remain a good guide for identifying autoimmune diseases.

Clinically, autoimmune diseases have been divided into **systemic** or '**non-organ-specific**' and '**organ-specific**' diseases. However, this categorisation is not absolute. Many autoimmune diseases have both organ-specific and non-organ-

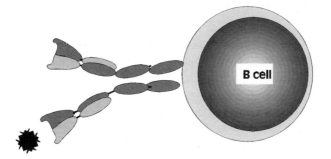

**B cell is stimulated by the major
antigenic determinant on a foreign antigen**

The same epitope is expressed on a self antigen

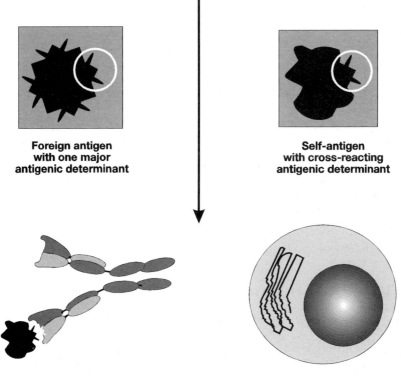

**Foreign antigen
with one major
antigenic determinant**

**Self-antigen
with cross-reacting
antigenic determinant**

**The resulting antibodies cross-react with the self-antigen
and thus bind to both the foreign and self antigens.**

Figure 9.1   The role of antigen mimicry in autoimmune disease.

If the major antigenic determinant of an infectious agent is similar antigenically to a self-antigen, then the response elicited by the micro-organism can result in an autoimmune response

Table 9.2 Examples of potential antigenic mimicry

Potential antigen mimicry	Disease association
Antibodies to measles virus cross-react with myelin basic protein	Multiple sclerosis
Antibodies to antigens from bacteria such as *Escherichia coli*, *Proteus vulgaris* and *Klebsiella pneumoniae* are thought to cross-react with acetylcholine receptors	Myasthenia gravis
Antibodies to a variety of phospholipids and bacteria may cross-react with DNA	Systemic lupus erythematosus (SLE)
Antibodies to *Klebsiella*-derived proteins show similarities to some anti-DNA antibodies	SLE and ankylosing spondylitis
Epstein–Barr virus nuclear antigen shares an antigen found in synovial membranes	Rheumatoid arthritis
An adenovirus type 12 protein shows structural similarities to α-gliadin in wheat	Coeliac disease

specific complications. Also, more than one type of disease may occur in the same individual.

The classical example of a non-organ-specific autoimmune disease is systemic lupus erythematosus (SLE), in which the autoimmune response is directed to a number of different tissue antigens. Such non-organ-specific diseases may develop as a result of an abnormal immune response to a single antigen which is expressed in many tissues.

There are a wide range of organ-specific autoimmune diseases, including Hashimoto's thyroiditis (the principal target organ being the thyroid) and insulin-dependent diabetes mellitus (pancreas).

IMMUNOPATHOLOGY OF AUTOIMMUNE DISEASES

Autoimmune diseases form a large, heterogeneous group with a wide variety of clinical signs and symptoms. Despite this disparity, the immunopathology of all these diseases may be considered to be the result of particular **hypersensitivity reactions**, each disease being the result of one or more type of response.

Type II Hypersensitivity Reactions

This type of reaction involves the interaction of an antibody with a cell surface antigen resulting in the formation of an immune complex which may activate complement or be a target for ADCC. In autoimmune diseases, the antibody recognises either a normal (usually sequestered) or modified (by viruses or chemicals) cellular self-antigen and the resulting immune complex stimulates a type II hypersensitivity response (Figure 9.2). The resultant tissue damage (pathology) gives rise to the signs and symptoms by which the disease is categorised.

Autoantibodies may also cause autoimmunity by interacting with cellular receptors, thus causing an abnormal expression of cellular activity, e.g. autoimmune haemolytic anaemia. In such a reaction, the autoantibody is not involved in an ADCC reaction.

Type III Hypersensitivity Reactions

Autoantibody may bind to self-antigens which are free in tissue fluids or in the general circulation. The resulting complexes are free to circulate throughout the body. However, they may become quite large (depending on the relative concentrations of antibody and antigen) and, therefore, insoluble. This results in their precipitation in the tissues and blood vessels. Particularly vulnerable are tissues with large filtering membranes, such as the kidneys, joints and choroid plexus, where the presence of immune complexes results in the activation of the complement cascade and inflammatory sequelae (Figure 9.3). As a direct consequence, localised cell death occurs and the function of the organ or tissues involved may be lost due to blockage of blood vessels by clot formation (e.g. vasculitis in systemic lupus erythematosus).

Type IV Hypersensitivity Reactions

T cells sensitised to self-antigens may cause tissue damage through the release of lymphokines which either directly damage the tissues (e.g. tumour necrosis factor) or attract inflammatory cells to the site which mediate the damage themselves.

THE IMMUNOLOGY OF AUTOIMMUNE DISEASE

Autoimmune diseases result from an abnormal immune response to self-antigens. In all these diseases there is a breakdown of normal regulatory mechanisms and a lack of **tolerance** to the self-antigens concerned. The complex immunological responses which occur in these diseases are responsible for the resulting pathology, and an understanding of these responses is vital for effective disease management.

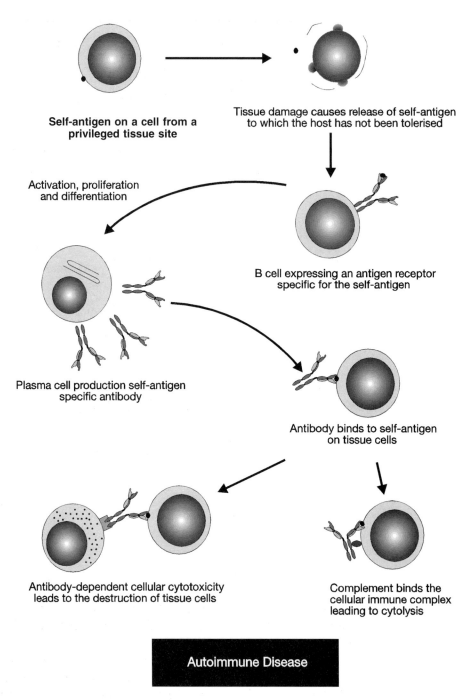

Self-antigen on a cell from a
privileged tissue site

Tissue damage causes release of self-antigen
to which the host has not been tolerised

Activation, proliferation
and differentiation

B cell expressing an antigen receptor
specific for the self-antigen

Plasma cell production self-antigen
specific antibody

Antibody binds to self-antigen
on tissue cells

Antibody-dependent cellular cytotoxicity
leads to the destruction of tissue cells

Complement binds the
cellular immune complex
leading to cytolysis

Autoimmune Disease

Figure 9.2   Type II hypersensitivity responses in autoimmunity.

Cells may express abnormal antigens or those to which the immune system is not normally exposed. When such exposure occurs, the resulting antibodies attach to the cell, forming an immune complex which may elicit a type II hypersensitivity response

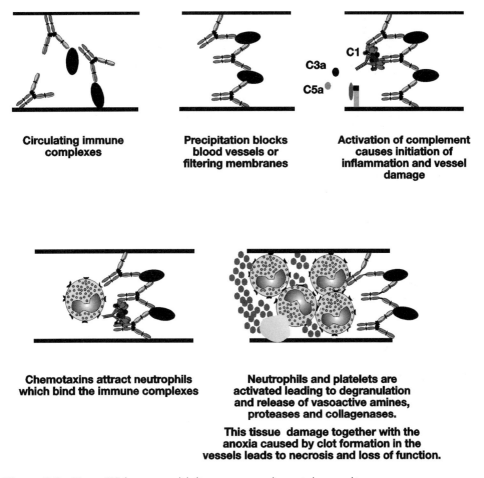

Circulating immune complexes

Precipitation blocks blood vessels or filtering membranes

Activation of complement causes initiation of inflammation and vessel damage

Chemotaxins attract neutrophils which bind the immune complexes

Neutrophils and platelets are activated leading to degranulation and release of vasoactive amines, proteases and collagenases.

This tissue damage together with the anoxia caused by clot formation in the vessels leads to necrosis and loss of function.

Figure 9.3 Type III hypersensitivity responses in autoimmunity.

Circulating immune complexes may precipitate in small blood vessels and cause complement activation. This results in inflammation which damages the vessel

Target Antigens

In many autoimmune diseases, the antigens which stimulate the disease or are the target of autoimmune attack are not clearly defined. There are some notable exceptions (Table 9.3).

Heat shock proteins (hsp) are a highly conserved group of antigens which have been implicated in the pathogenesis of a number of autoimmune diseases. When cells are stressed, the heat shock proteins are produced preferentially and confer some protective effect on the stressed cells. They are so highly conserved that even bacteria produce these proteins and they show a high degree of homology to those produced by animals of various species. These proteins are grouped into families according to their molecular weight. Cell surface

Table 9.3   Target antigens involved in autoimmune diseases

Disease	Target antigens/Potential target antigens
Myasthenia gravis	Acetylcholine receptor
Primary biliary cirrhosis	Mitochondrial enzymes of the 2-oxo-acid dehydrogenase family
Autoimmune thyroid disease	Thyroid-stimulating hormone receptor, thyroid peroxidase and thyroglobulin
Systemic lupus erythematosus	Double-stranded DNA

expression of hsp 90 has been shown to be increased in about one fifth of patients with systemic lupus erythematosus (particularly on B cells and CD4+ T cells). In contrast, hsp 65 levels are increased in patients with rheumatoid arthritis.

Non-specific Immunity in Autoimmune Disease

In recent years, a model has been proposed which propounds that **non-specific immune mechanisms** (i.e. those which are not dependent upon specific recognition of antigen) are involved in the initiation of autoimmune diseases such as multiple sclerosis, rheumatoid arthritis, thyroiditis and diabetes. This model, the **REGA** (**r**emnant **e**pitope **g**enerates **a**utoantigen) **model**, proposes that the disease is triggered by an agent which induces the production of disease-enhancing cytokines, which in turn stimulate the production of a range of other cytokines, including chemokines for monocytes and neutrophils. These cytokines stimulate resident macrophages to produce proteinases and activate latent metalloproteinases. This has been shown to lead directly to demyelination in multiple sclerosis. These proteinases cause the production of a large number of peptides from myelin basic protein which may be processed and presented to T cells. This implies that the specific cell-mediated autoimmunity develops at a relatively late stage of disease onset.

   Further indirect evidence for a role of non-specific mechanisms in the development of autoimmunity is provided by the observation that cytokines which suppress proteinase activity, e.g. IFNα and IFNβ, predominate in the remission phase of multiple sclerosis and rheumatoid arthritis.

Macrophages in Autoimmune Disease

Mononuclear phagocytes play a central role in immunity. Not only do they fulfil a role in non-specific immunity through the phagocytosis of opsonised particles but also they are instrumental in controlling antigen-specific responses through antigen processing and presentation to lymphocytes.

Mononuclear Phagocytes in Non-specific Immunity

Clearance, in vivo, of antibody-sensitised red blood cells has been reported to be decreased in humans with autoimmune diseases. The persistence of immune complexes may contribute to the pathology observed and may be the result of defective phagocytic cell function or be the cause of it by blocking Fc receptors. However, studies have shown that the number of Fcγ receptors on mononuclear cells are normal or increased in patients with systemic lupus erythematosus (a disease in which circulating immune complexes are typically present) and there is no correlation between the level of circulating immune complexes and the magnitude of the clearance defect.

Another receptor which is involved in phagocytosis is the C3b receptor, the expression of which has been reported to be decreased in patients with systemic lupus erythematosus and rheumatoid arthritis. Regardless of what causes the change in expression of these opsonin receptors (both FcγR and C3R), the result is likely to manifest as a decrease in clearance of immune complexes, leading to an increase in their deposition in tissues (such as the kidney) which may complicate the clinical course of the disease (e.g. glomerular nephritis).

As mentioned earlier, macrophages have been implicated in the initiation of autoimmune diseases through the production of disease-promoting cytokines and proteinases.

Mononuclear Phagocytes in Specific Immunity

Changes in the cell surface expression of the MHC Class II gene product DR have been recorded in both non-organ-specific and organ-specific autoimmune diseases. For example, epithelial cells in the thyroid of many patients with Graves' disease show high levels of HLA-DR, an antigen not usually found on normal thyroid epithelium. Also, abnormal presentation of foreign antigens (resulting from an unusual association between an antigen such as a drug or micro-organism and HLA-DR) has been implicated as a cause of systemic lupus erythematosus. Such an association would appear as an altered self-antigen, thus providing a new epitope which may be recognised, and reacted to, by helper T cells. As a consequence, the latter produce lymphokines which stimulate the differentiation and proliferation of activated, self-reactive, B cells.

The mechanisms which cause the abnormal expression of DR antigens have not been determined. It is known that interferon induces HLA-DR expression on epithelial cells and that viruses may induce the production of interferon. Thus, it has been suggested that such an infection could induce HLA-DR expression on thyroid epithelium, allowing antigen presentation by cells not usually involved in this process. This may therefore increase the chance of unusual presentation of self-antigens and recognition by T cells, leading to the development of autoimmune disease.

ROLE OF T CELLS IN AUTOIMMUNE DISEASE

The Thymus

The thymus plays a vital role in the development of self-tolerance, and thus abnormalities affecting the development or functioning of the thymus may contribute to the development of autoimmune diseases. For example, a variety of thymic abnormalities have been reported in systemic lupus erythematosus, but it is unclear whether these are causative, or sequelae, of the disease.

The TCR Repertoire in Autoimmune Diseases

In recent years, evidence has been accumulated which indicates the restricted usage of particular TCR V region genes. In rheumatoid arthritis, the majority of T cells in the synovial fluid appear to express the Vβ8 (variable region gene number 8 of the β chain of the TCR) TCR gene product, suggesting a restricted repertoire in autoimmune disease. However, many other Vβ and Jβ gene products were also detected, indicating that the autoimmune response is not restricted to one or two T cell clones. Indeed, further studies have indicated that any restriction of the repertoire is limited to the genes of the junctional region of the TCR on CD8+ cells.

In myasthenia gravis, patients have been shown to have increased expression of the Vβ5.1 and Vβ8 genes in the peripheral blood and on mature thymocytes but not on precursor thymic cells. This suggests that these patients may exhibit an altered thymic selection process.

T Helper Cells

Self-tolerance is maintained even though autoreactive B cells may be present. This is thought to be because T cell tolerance is long-lasting and therefore autoreactive B cells lack the T cell help they require. This T cell control may be demonstrated in vitro by the use of B cell mitogens or purified lymphokines, which eliminate the need for T cell help. In vivo, T cell maintenance of tolerance may be overcome in a number of ways (Table 9.4).

T Suppressor Cells

In many autoimmune diseases, changes in the number and functional activity of Ts cells have been reported. However, many of these observations have been

Table 9.4 Mechanisms involved in the breakdown of T cell self-tolerance

Cause of abnormal self-antigen production	Effect
Abnormal synthesis or processing of self-antigen	Self-antigen with novel antigenic determinants
Drugs	e.g. aspirin may combine with proteins in the tissues, resulting in a new antigenic complex
Viruses or drugs	Novel association of different proteins (either self or viral), resulting in new antigenic determinants
Antigenic mimicry	Non-self, cross-reactive antigens stimulate T cells, which may then recognise self-antigens

contradictory and their significance in organ-specific disease is unclear, since only a very few Ts cells are involved in maintaining tolerance to any one antigen. Elimination of these would not be detectable as a statistically significant decrease in the total number of CD8 + cells in the blood. Such a decrease would have to be more generalised, and it is difficult to see how this might result in an organ-specific disease, although it may be important in non-organ-specific diseases such as SLE.

B Cells in Autoimmune Disease

Abnormal B cell activity is common in autoimmune diseases and is typified by the production of polyclonal antibodies, many of which react with self-antigens. Such autoantibody production may be a primary cause of disease or may result from abnormal T cell control. It may also affect the normal function of T cells, thus causing an acceleration of the disease. In myasthenia gravis, antibodies to the muscle nicotinic acetylcholine receptor (AChR) are responsible for the majority of the clinical symptoms observed. Other antibodies which recognise presynaptic membrane proteins or sarcoplasmic membrane proteins are thought to play a role in the pathogenesis of the disease, particularly in patients lacking anti-AChR antibodies.

Abnormal B cell activity may be the result of genetic (e.g. certain autoreactive B cells may be extremely sensitive to selected stimuli, due to their genetic make-up) or mitogenic (e.g. either endogenous or exogenous mitogens stimulate the formation of autoantibodies) factors, but both depend upon the presence of self-reactive B cells. However, such cells are normally eliminated during fetal development; their persistence results from the differences in tolerance induction in T and B cells. Self-antigens present in low concentrations may cause tolerance induction in T cells but fail to cause elimination of B cells which recognise them. These self-reactive B cells may be activated by substances which interact with them directly (e.g. T-independent antigens from bacteria and viruses), resulting in the production of autoantibodies. However, since such **polyclonal stimulators** usually induce the production of low-affinity, IgM autoantibodies and the tissue damage seen in autoimmune diseases usually results from the action of IgG autoantibodies, it is unlikely that polyclonal activators alone can cause chronic disease.

B Cell Differentiation and Proliferation

Resting B cells need at least three signals to stimulate their proliferation and differentiation into antibody-producing cells (Figure 9.4). Depending upon the nature of the stimulus, the signals come from (i) recognition by T cells of antigen in association with HLA-DR on B cells or cross-linking of mIg on B cells by a T-independent antigen; (ii) recognition of antigen by mIg on B cells; (iii) association of T cell-derived lymphokines (e.g. IL-2, IL-4, IL-5, IL-6) with appropriate receptors on the B cells.

The pathology seen in autoimmune diseases may reflect abnormalities in B cell signal requirements, regulation of lymphokine production, or B cell responses to lymphokines.

In myasthenia gravis, anti-AChR antibodies are thought to cause pathology through the degradation of the receptor, either by cross-linking or through complement-mediated lysis of post-synaptic membranes; they do not commonly affect signal transduction through blocking the cholinergic binding site. The antibodies produced usually do not recognise a single antigenic epitope, and even those which do, do not show restricted gene usage. This suggests that myasthenia gravis is not the result of the escape from tolerance of a single self-reactive clone. Also, the poor correlation between anti-AChR antibody levels and disease progression suggests that only some clones are pathogenic.

These may result in hypergammaglobulinaemia (abnormally high serum levels of immunoglobulin), autoantibody production, the preferential production of pathogenic subclasses of autoantibodies or a generalised autoimmune disease such as SLE.

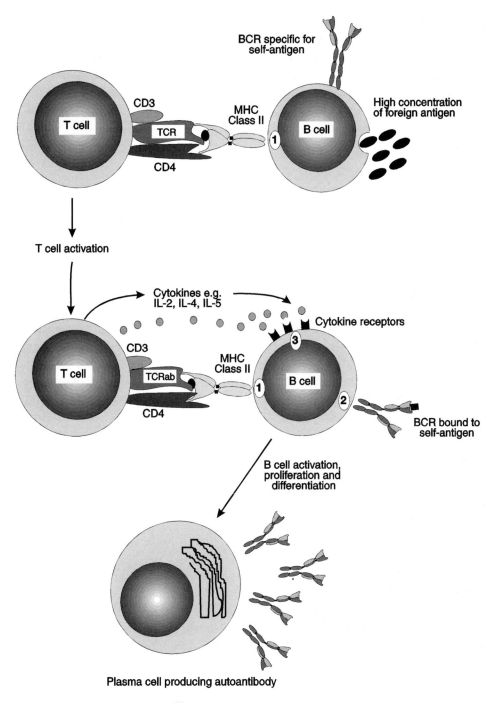

Figure 9.4   Production of autoantibody by B cells.

B cells which recognise self-antigen may be stimulated to differentiate into plasma cells producing autoantibody after receiving help from appropriately stimulated T cells

Table 9.5   Lymphokine abnormalities in autoimmune diseases

Lymphokine	Disease
Defective IL-2 production	Systemic lupus erythematosus and rheumatoid arthritis
Defective IL-1 production	Systemic lupus erythematosus and rheumatoid arthritis
Qualitative and quantitative abnormalities in interferon	Systemic autoimmune diseases
High levels of acid-labile IFNα	Systemic lupus erythematosus

Lymphokine Defects

As with all clinical studies in humans, data concerning lymphokine production in patients with autoimmune diseases are often controversial or inconclusive. Such studies may be influenced by a number of factors, including genetic factors, hormonal changes, diurnal variation, disease type and other infectious or medical complications, including therapy. Thus, the relevance of abnormalities observed in serum lymphokine levels to the disease process is difficult to interpret, especially in organ-specific diseases, where serum levels may not reflect those occurring within the affected tissues. Some accepted observations are listed in Table 9.5.

LEARNING OUTCOMES

This chapter has been designed to help you understand the importance of self-tolerance with respect to health. Autoimmune disease results from a breakdown of those mechanisms which normally prevent the body from reacting to self-antigens. Such a breakdown can result in severely debilitating or even fatal disease. Any tissue in the body may be the target for an autoimmune disease. The range of tissues affected depends upon the specific self-antigen being recognised and its distribution; if the antigen is expressed in a number of different tissues or organs, the disease will be widely disseminated; if it is only expressed in one particular organ, an organ-specific disease will result.

Chapter 10

Mucosal Immunity

LEARNING OBJECTIVES

The major internal regions of the body which connect with the exterior are lined by **mucosal membranes**. With the exception of the skin, which is a horny, keratinised surface and relatively impervious to micro-organisms, the mucosae are the major area through which micro-organisms can enter the body. In addition, because they are moist, warm and usually lubricated by nutrient-containing fluid, the mucosal membranes form an excellent environment for promoting the growth of bacteria. The mucosal immune system has evolved to protect these regions from infection. It comprises the **lymphoid tissues** associated with the mucosae of the **respiratory, gastrointestinal** and **urogenital tracts**.

The purpose of this chapter is to introduce you to the structure and organisation of the mucosal immune system and to give you an understanding of its importance in maintaining health and in immunisation.

THE STRUCTURE OF THE MUCOSAL IMMUNE SYSTEM

The largest part of the mucosal immune system is made up of the immunological tissue found in the gastrointestinal tract. Its importance can be put into context by considering the fact that it contains as much lymphoid tissue as the spleen, one of the major lymphoid organs.

The mucosal immune system can be subdivided into the **organised tissues** (where immunologically active cells can encounter antigen and initiate the immune response) and **diffuse lymphoid tissue** (in which effector cells perform their functions, e.g. secretion of antigen-specific antibody). The organised tissues (known as the **gut-associated lymphoid tissues** or **GALT** and **bronchus-associated lymphoid tissues** or **BALT**) consist of the mucosal follicles. The diffuse lymphoid tissue, as its name suggest, has no organised structure and includes all those immunologically relevant cells which are scattered throughout the lamina propria of mucosal membranes. Some of the cells which are stimulated by antigen (sensitised) in the mucosal follicles develop into memory cells and move ('home') to the diffuse lymphoid tissues, where they are likely to be re-exposed to their stimulating antigen. After homing to the diffuse tissues, most of the memory B cells develop into IgA-producing cells.

Organised Mucosal Lymphoid Tissue

The organised lymphoid tissue of the mucosae form aggregates which are different from those of the systemic lymphoid system. Rather than reaching the mucosal aggregates through the blood or lymphatic circulations, antigen arrives through the epithelial cells. Those which transport the antigen are specialised, flattened epithelial cells called M cells (membranous cells) which cover the lymphoid aggregates.

Initially, antigen binds to the M cell surface, presumably through particular binding sites (although these have yet to be identified). It is taken into pinocytic vesicles in which it is transported through the cell, and is finally released in an unaltered form into the sub-epithelial area. Neither binding nor uptake is totally indiscriminate; there is some evidence that the transport of bacteria by M cells is inhibited by specific antibodies which may interact with bacterial determinants necessary for binding to M cells. The ability to be taken up by M cells may have an impact on the virulence of an organism. The binding of viruses to M cells and their uptake by them may be an obligate means of entry and therefore a positive virulence factor, whereas uptake leading to antibody formation and immune elimination of the organism has a negative impact on virulence.

M cells do not express MHC Class II antigens and therefore are not capable of classical antigen presentation. By contrast, the epithelial cells do express Class II antigens (expression being enhanced during inflammation) and are capable of antigen presentation (at least in vitro).

Dome Area

Immediately beneath the epithelium of the lymphoid aggregates is the dome area which is rich in MHC Class II antigen-bearing cells such as macrophages, dendritic cells and B cells. Thus, this region is geared to antigen presentation following exposure of the mucosa to antigens. The dome areas also contain many T cells and although most of these cells are CD4+, a number lack both CD4 and CD8. This latter population may be **contrasuppressor cells**.

Follicular Zone

Beneath the dome area is the region known as the follicular zone, where the **germinal centres** are located. Hence, B cells predominate, although T cells are scattered throughout the region. The B cells are highly differentiated mIgD+ and, unlike other germinal centre B cells, up to 40% are mIgA+. Although providing an environment for the development of mIgA+ B cells, the mucosal follicle lacks IgA-secreting plasma cells, presumably because the B cells leave the follicle before differentiating into plasma cells.

Between the follicles, the tissues are rich in T cells and the majority of the mucosal lymphoid aggregate CD8+ T cells are found here.

Diffuse Mucosal Lymphoid Tissue

The diffuse lymphoid tissues of the mucosae consist of the **intraepithelial lymphocyte (IEL)** compartment and the **lamina propria lymphocyte (LPL)** compartment.

Intraepithelial Lymphocytes

Intraepithelial lymphocytes are found above the basement membrane, distributed amongst the epithelial cells. They are phenotypically heterogeneous, but the majority of T cells present are CD3+, CD2+, CD8+. Recently, it has been shown that proliferation of these cells can be stimulated via the CD2 molecule but not the T cell receptor.

> Studies with mice suggest that IELs have specialised effector functions which include natural killer cell activity, antigen-specific cellular cytotoxicity and secretion of interferon-gamma (IFNγ), which causes an increase in MHC Class II antigen and γ/δ T cell receptor expression on epithelial cells.

Lamina Propria Lymphocytes

Lamina propria lymphocytes are found beneath the epithelial layer in the lamina propria and comprise roughly equal numbers of B and T cells. The majority of B cells are mIgA+ but, in order of decreasing frequency, mIgM+, mIgG+ and mIgE+ B cells are also found.

Lamina propria T cells have been shown to contain mRNA for interleukin-2 (IL-2) and its receptor (IL-2R), and for IFNγ. These cells also show increased expression of MHC Class II antigens and the IL-2R. CD4+ T cells from the lamina propria respond to specific antigens by secreting cytokines rather than by proliferating, suggesting that such cells are a type of memory T cell.

Lamina Propria Macrophages

Cells which have the morphology of typical macrophages are found concentrated in the more superficial parts of the mucosae, just below the epithelium. In the lamina propria, a high proportion of macrophages express MHC Class II antigens and other phenotypic markers associated with activation, indicating that they are in a more highly activated state than the corresponding cells in other lymphoid areas. Not only are these macrophages likely to be important in non-specific host defence, but they also produce cytokines, such as IL-1 and IL-6, which stimulate the **specific immune response**.

Lamina Propria NK and Lymphokine-activated Killer (LAK) Cells

Natural killer (NK) cells which are CD16+ and/or CD56+ are found only occasionally in the lamina propria and their activity is difficult to demonstrate in lamina propria-derived lymphocyte populations. By contrast, cells with lymphokine-activated killer function are easily demonstrated in these populations. LAK cells are either CD8+ T cells or NK cells that exert antigen non-specific cytotoxicity when exposed to IL-2.

Lamina Propria Mast Cells

The mucosae are rich in mast cell precursors, which rapidly differentiate into mature mast cells when they are appropriately stimulated. These play a vital role in the non-specific immune response by stimulating **inflammation**.

IMMUNOGLOBULINS AND MUCOSAL IMMUNITY

Immunoglobulin A

The production of IgA is one of the distinguishing characteristics of the mucosal immune response. The advantages obtained by the secretion of IgA in such tissues derive from a number of unique properties that allow IgA to function more efficiently than other immunoglobulins in the mucosal environment.

Regulation of IgA Synthesis at Mucosal Sites

Unlike in other lymphoid tissue, the B cells of the mucosal follicles preferentially produce IgA. Cells obtained from such tissue (e.g. from the Peyer's patches of the gut) have been shown (in vitro) to induce IgA secretion by B cells. The cells causing this isotype switch were T cells, but it is possible that other cells such as mucosal macrophages and stromal cells may also play a role. The signals for isotype switching are probably provided by cytokines. However, neither IL-4 nor IL-5 can perform this function alone. It is possible that they act in synergy with other factors.

B cells in mucosal tissue are affected by signals which favour the terminal differentiation of IgA-secreting B cells. These signals are derived from FcαR+ T cells, which are thought to release IgA-binding factors which act on mIgA-positive B cells. In addition, evidence suggests that some T cells secrete IL-5 which, in concert with other cytokines such as IL-6, preferentially stimulates mIgA-positive B cell differentiation. Thus, the secretion of IgA by mucosal tissues may reflect the selective distribution of these T cells in such tissues.

Production of Other Immunoglobulins in the Mucosa

Apart from IgA, other immunoglobulins play a role in mucosal immunity. IgM, which can be transported across the epithelial cell layer, is produced in physiologically significant quantities by the mucosae. Its importance is demonstrated by the fact that it can provide **mucosal immunity** in persons with selective IgA deficiency. By contrast, IgG production is quite low in most mucosal areas. It cannot be transported across the epithelium but does have a role to play in the lungs where it is found in the pulmonary secretions, probably entering by passive diffusion.

Although IgE is synthesised in the mucosae, IgE-secreting B cells do not show preferential localisation and, indeed, their number is as small as it is in other tissues. However, mucosal IgE is particularly apparent during parasitic infection or allergic reactions.

THE MUCOSAE AND THEIR ROLE IN IMMUNITY

The mucosal immune system has a number of distinct features. In addition to the preferential secretion of IgA and the presence of T cells which influence its IgA production by B cells, the mucosae have a characteristic cell-trafficking system whereby cells, initially stimulated in the mucosal follicles (**mucosal inductive sites**), migrate to the diffuse, sub-epithelial lymphoid tissues (**mucosal effector sites**). The latter effectively results in the partitioning of the mucosal cells from the systemic circulation, making the mucosal immune system almost independent of the rest of the immune system.

Functions

The majority of potential pathogens first gain access to the body through the mucosal membranes which cover the surface of the gut, the lungs and the urogenital tract. Thus, the mucosal immune system provides a primary line of defence which is helped by a number of non-immunological factors such as the normal mucosal flora of the host, secretions (including mucus, gastric acid and intestinal bile), involuntary movement (such as peristalsis, ciliary action, coughing, sneezing and defecating) and chemicals such as lactoferrin and spermine. However, these non-immunological factors are not very effective alone, since immunodeficient patients often present with mucosal infections (e.g. oral candidiasis in patients with the acquired immune deficiency syndrome — AIDS).

Many antigens which come in contact with the mucosal immune system derive from food or the normal microbial flora. It would not be appropriate for an immune response to be mounted to such antigens, particularly a systemic response. Therefore, the mucosal immune system exhibits a state of **unresponsiveness (tolerance)** to such antigens and is adapted to prevent the

> Studies in sheep have shown that the cell turnover in Peyer's patches is vast, cells showing a high rate of mortality. It has been suggested that this may represent a process of negative clonal selection, as in the thymus; surviving cells show tolerance to antigens derived from food and normal microbial flora.

exposure of the systemic immune system to them. In addition, T cells of the mucosal immune system **downregulate** systemic immune responses to antigens which cross the mucosal barrier, the antigens being removed via the **liver.**

Mucosal unresponsiveness to oral antigens is both B and T cell-mediated, although the same degree of unresponsiveness may not be exhibited to all antigens. The lack of response to antigenic stimulation in the mucosal follicles may be due, in part, to the stimulation of antigen-specific suppressor T cells as demonstrated in the Peyer's patches of the gut. This may be enhanced by the presence of antigen-non-specific suppressor cells.

Mucosal Homing

A characteristic feature of the mucosal immune system is the **homing** capability of cells developing in the mucosal follicles. This acts to limit and focus the mucosal immune response to mucosal tissues. Characteristically, T and B cells stimulated in the mesenteric (gut-associated) or bronchial lymph nodes undergo blast transformation and migrate to the lymphoid tissue associated with the mucosae. Between 70 and 90% of the B cells have undergone isotype switching to IgA. The T cell blasts localise in the lamina propria and the IEL compartment; however, these represent only a small proportion of the T cells recirculating in the mucosal immune system. Memory B cells and T cells which arise in the mucosal follicles also recirculate.

Antigenic stimulation at one site in the mucosal immune system leads to the appearance of reactive cells at other non-exposed mucosal sites. This suggests that cell migration is not directed by antigen. Once the cells have reached the tissues, they are stimulated by antigen to proliferate and thus become fixed at this site. In this way, antigen-specific responses are enhanced in areas that have been previously exposed to antigen.

The process of mucosal homing is thought to be initiated through the interaction of specific homing receptors on lymphocytes from the Peyer's patches and their ligands (addressins) on endothelial cells. Following this contact, the cells penetrate the endothelium, gaining access to the mucosal tissues. Thus, homing of lymphocytes to the lymphoid tissues of the mucosae probably reflects the selective expression of homing receptors by these cells.

MUCOSAL IMMUNITY AND VACCINATION

Since the majority of the body is covered by a layer of keratinous skin, the majority of pathogenic micro-organisms cause infection after entering the body via the mucosal membranes which line the respiratory, gastrointestinal and urogenital tracts. In order to control or prevent such infections, it is necessary to understand the way in which immunity may be induced at the mucosal surface.

The mucosal immune system can be divided into discrete inductive sites, where antigens are processed, and presented to B and T cells (the organised mucosal tissues), and effector sites, where the mucosal immune response actually occurs (the diffuse mucosal tissues). Memory B cells migrate to the mucosal effector tissues, where they differentiate into IgA-secreting plasma cells, a characteristic of these tissues. In addition, it has been proposed that antigen-specific Th cells and even CD8 + cytotoxic T lymphocytes can cycle from inductive to mucosal effector sites; all these elements (including memory B cells) comprise the **common mucosal immune system** (CMIS).

As might be expected, the gut mucosal immune system is vital to the defence of the host against many pathogenic organisms, especially those causing enteric infections which are accompanied by diarrhoea. Vaccination against such infections has largely been unsuccessful (when compared with vaccination against systemic infections), probably due to a lack of understanding of the peculiar requirements for inducing protective, local, immune responses at mucosal surfaces. However, it has been shown that secretory IgA (sIgA) antibodies generated in the mucosal tissue of the gut, airways or urogenital tracts can provide protection against infections in these sites.

From what we have learnt already, it is likely that immunity at mucosal surfaces (which is largely dependent upon the production of antigen-specific IgA) would require a Th2-type response. Indeed, some studies have shown that oral immunisation preferentially induces such a response and leads to antigen-specific IgA responses in mucosal effector sites. The antigen-specific Th2 cells are probably induced in the Peyer's patches of the gut (inductive site) and migrate to effector sites, where they regulate the activation and differentiation of antigen-specific mIgA + B cells through the production of cytokines such as IL-5 and IL-6. These observations would suggest that in order to provide the appropriate protection, oral vaccines should be designed to ensure the induction of a Th2 cell response in appropriate mucosal sites. Indeed, it has been shown that such vaccines must induce a Th2 response in both inductive and effector sites of the mucosae in order to induce a protective sIgA response. This means that care must be taken when delivering antigens by live vectors such as *Salmonella typhi* which typically activate a Th1 response preferentially (as is seen with many intracellular pathogens) and would thus fail to induce the Th2 response required for efficient sIgA production.

Recently, an effective oral vaccine against cholera has been developed and vaccines to other infectious agents are being developed (e.g. *Shigella*, enterotoxigenic *E. coli* and enteroviruses). However, these vaccines require repeated injection of large antigen doses to produce a protective response, making the current protocols limited in application. However, with the development of new techniques for enhancing delivery of antigen to the mucosal immune system and of adjuvants with the ability to stimulate it, the potential exists to develop vaccines against not only gut infections, but also those affecting the respiratory and urogenital tracts.

LEARNING OUTCOMES

The mucosae provide a unique environment for the development of immunity. Since many infectious agents are first encountered by the mucosal immune system, it plays a vital role in maintaining health and preventing disease. Also, when developing effective vaccines, it is vital to understand how the mucosal immune system responds to antigenic stimulation. This chapter should have given you an insight into these mechanisms and equipped you with the basic knowledge you need to understand the references cited in the Further Reading.

Chapter 11

Immunity to Infection

LEARNING OBJECTIVES

Every day we are exposed to an enormous number of bacteria, viruses, fungi and parasites. However, most of us are usually quite healthy. Relatively few of these organisms cause infection but when they do so, they may cause tissue damage in the host. If these organisms are allowed to grow unchecked, they will cause the death of the host either directly or indirectly. However, most infections do not have such a terminal outcome and in people who are generally healthy, infection is usually confined and any tissue damage easily repaired. This 'damage limitation' is brought about by the cellular and chemical components of the immune system acting together to limit the spread of the infection, kill the micro-organisms and repair the tissue damage.

The ability of different organisms to cause disease (their **pathogenicity**) varies greatly and is related to how easily they can be controlled by the immune system. The latter comprises a group of mechanisms which may be called sequentially into play, gradually increasing the overall effectiveness of the immune response. For ease of description these mechanisms have been divided into two basic groups: the **non-specific** or **innate** and the **specific** or **adaptive immune responses**.

The purpose of this chapter is to bring together all the information presented in the previous chapters to illustrate the role of the immune system in immunity to infection. We shall examine the relative contributions of both non-specific and specific defence mechanisms in overcoming infection. It must be remembered that these two groups generally do not act independently but show areas of overlap. The innate immune response is non-specific; the cellular and chemical events which occur may do so in response to any micro-organism or to tissue damage. These mechanisms do not specifically recognise the causative agent; they merely react to the stimulus that has upset the normal situation. By contrast, the adaptive immune response is designed to specifically recognise the causative agent and to eliminate it.

THE INNATE IMMUNE SYSTEM

In order for an organism to cause infection, it must first overcome a number of physical barriers which are often considered to be part of the innate immune system. These barriers — the skin, the respiratory epithelium, the gastrointestinal epithelium, etc. — are largely non-specific and non-immunological, but play a vital role in host defence (Figure 11.1).

The Skin

The skin provides a horny, keratinised layer that is not breached easily and hence provides a very efficient barrier against microbial invasion. Its dry nature, the presence of competing micro-organisms and various chemical secretions all combine to prevent colonisation by potentially pathogenic micro-organisms. The skin and sweat have a number of substances which are inhibitory or toxic to bacteria and fungi. These include a high content of fatty acids and the enzyme **lysozyme**.

The Mucosae

Many pathogens cause infection by gaining entry to the body through the mucosal membranes lining the gut, lungs and urogenital tracts. The epithelial cells which make up these membranes are coated with a mucus layer which helps to prevent micro-organisms attaching to the cell surface. Some mucous membranes have cilia, tiny, hair-like projections, the movement of which wafts any organisms trapped in the mucus out of the body. This process may be accelerated by reflex actions such as coughing or sneezing, which propel entrapped organisms out of the body at great speed. In addition, infection may be limited by the short half-life of intestinal epithelial cells (approximately 30 hours). If invading micro-organisms happen to attach to an epithelial cell as it is shed (**desquamation**), infection is prevented.

Various chemical substances secreted by the mucosae also aid in protection against infection. These include **lactoferrin**, an iron-binding protein which sequesters free iron such that the concentration falls below that necessary for bacterial growth.

Protective Chemicals

Lysozyme

Probably the most ubiquitous antibacterial substance formed at body surfaces is lysozyme. This enzyme is present in tears, saliva, sweat and many other

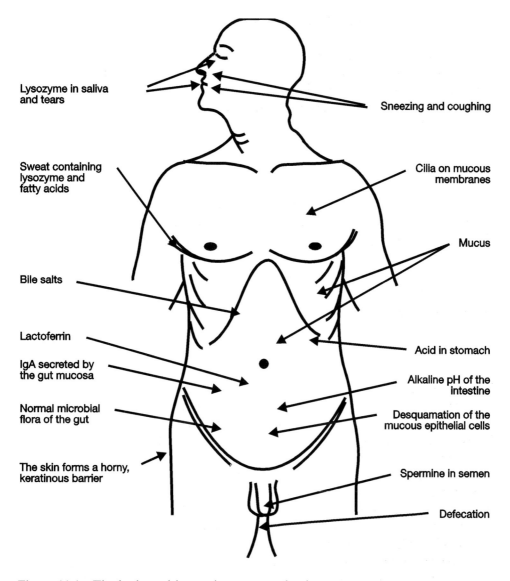

Figure 11.1   The body and innate immune mechanisms

mucosal secretions. It is bactericidal for many Gram-positive bacteria, where it destroys the integrity of the cell wall by disrupting the N-acetyl muramic acid-N-acetylglucosamine linkages.

The highly acidic contents of the stomach are enough to kill most gastrointestinal pathogens. Organisms surviving this environment then have to face the alkaline nature of the intestine.

Complement

Complement acts by inactivating micro-organisms and by enhancing their phagocytosis (**opsonisation**). Breakdown products induce **vasodilation** and are **chemoattractants**. Thus, complement plays an important role in **inflammation**. Although the **classical pathway** generally requires the presence of **immune complexes** for its activation, the **alternative complement pathway** can be stimulated to kill some Gram-negative bacteria and to inactivate certain viruses in the absence of antibodies. Early in infection, prior to synthesis of specific antibodies, the ability of the alternative complement pathway to non-specifically opsonise or kill certain bacteria may be critical to recovery from infections.

In some fungal infections, complement has a vital role to play. Certain fungi bind fragments of C3 which may allow attachment and phagocytosis by polymorphonuclear leukocytes; for example, C3bi, C3d and C3d,g bind to *Cryptococcus neoformans*. However, whilst this is essential for the phagocytosis of encapsulated cryptococci, on its own it is not sufficient, since some species which bind these fragments are resistant to phagocytosis. Other fungi may bind directly to **complement receptors** on the cell surface (e.g. *Candida albicans*).

Defensins

In recent years, a large number of small peptides have been identified which exhibit antimicrobial activity. These **defensins** are widely distributed, are usually cationic, are of molecular mass 3–4 kDa and contain a high number of cysteine residues. The ability of these peptides to disrupt biological membranes may be important for their mechanism of action. The granules in neutrophils are the richest sources of defensins in humans (they are the most abundant protein in azurophilic granules) and comprise about 5% of the total protein in these cells.

Classical defensins have a triple-stranded structure and those from humans dimerise in crystalline form, the molecules associating in apposition. The antimicrobial activity of defensins is thought to result from their ability to accumulate as multimers in the lipid bilayer of target cells in such a way that they form **cyclic peptides**. These form channels in lipid membranes, increasing membrane permeability by a charge- or voltage-dependent mechanism.

Defensins are effective at very low levels (typically 10–100 μg/ml) against Gram-positive and Gram-negative bacteria, mycobacteria, fungi and enveloped viruses, including HIV. Classical defensins permeabilise both outer and inner membranes of Gram-negative bacteria. Their importance in protection against infection is exemplified by individuals who lack them. Patients with a rare, congenital, specific granule deficiency suffer from frequent infections caused by common bacteria.

Defensins and other antimicrobial peptides are relatively ineffective against pathogenic strains of *Salmonella typhimurium*. Interestingly, strains in which mutations have occurred that increase the susceptibility of these organisms to defensins in vitro, generally exhibit diminished virulence in a murine model.

Natural Antibodies

The antibodies which are found in the serum and make up the serum globulins are known as **natural antibodies**. These are produced generally by B cell clones with unmutated germ line genes and express low affinity for many self-antigens and foreign antigens. A major characteristic of these natural antibodies is a high degree of connectivity. Their biological role is not well documented but they could play a role in neutralising toxic metabolites, in the early stages of defence against micro-organisms, or in the elimination of old or transformed cells.

The Role of Normal Body Flora

Most body surfaces that are exposed to the environment are colonised by bacteria and fungi which are non-pathogenic or only weakly pathogenic. These are collectively known as the **normal flora**. These micro-organisms compete for attachment sites with other potentially pathogenic organisms and prevent them colonising the body surfaces. Also, they condition their local environment, which may make it unsuitable for the growth of pathogenic organisms whilst supporting the growth of the normal commensals. The normal flora clearly has a protective role to play since, if its balance is upset, e.g. in the gut by antibiotic treatment, patients become much more susceptible to infection by enteric pathogens such as *Shigella* sp. and *Salmonella* sp.

The protection afforded by the normal flora may result from competition with potential pathogens for nutrients or for receptor sites on epithelial cells, or may result from the secretion of toxic substances such as short-chain fatty acids which are secreted by intestinal anaerobes.

The Role of the Innate Immune System in Invasion

In spite of the physical and chemical barriers described above, potentially pathogenic organisms may invade the body. This arises because micro-organisms have evolved to avoid aspects of the immune response. For example,

Gram-positive organisms may be lysed by the action of lysozyme, but Gram-negative organisms have a **lipopolysaccharide membrane** which protects them from the action of this enzyme.

Invasion involves several steps, the first of which is attachment. Before organisms can invade the body, they must attach in some way to a cell. If you think about the common forms of infection, most of them occur through mucosal surfaces, and many bacteria are able to adhere to these surfaces using pili, proteinaceous projections which bind to receptors on the cell surface. Similarly, viruses must adhere to receptors on the surface of their target cells. This adherence may be prevented by the IgA present in mucosal secretions. However, certain organisms can overcome this blockage by secreting enzymes which destroy the IgA (e.g. *Gonococcus* sp.).

Once an organism has successfully made an attachment and has invaded the body, the innate immune response involves the collaboration of cells (the polymorphonuclear leukocytes), serum proteins (complement, acute-phase proteins, the clotting cascade, the kinin system) and a number of chemicals released from cells which affect the blood vessels (vasoactive amines). As a result of invasion and/or tissue damage, events occur which collectively form the **inflammatory response** (Chapter 5). These are designed to limit the infection/damage to the site of origin.

Fever

An increase in body temperature (fever) in response to infection occurs in humans and many other animals. This effect is caused by a combination of lymphokines, including IL-1, IL-6 and tumour necrosis factor (TNF). Although fever may be life-threatening to the host, it is beneficial in that many micro-organisms are sensitive to even very small temperature rises. This will not necessarily kill the organisms but will slow their growth enough to allow the immune response to eliminate the infection. Also, many of the protective responses in the host are more efficient at temperatures which are slightly greater than normal body temperature.

Cells Involved in Innate Immunity

Phagocytic Cells

Phagocytic cells include neutrophils and eosinophils (polymorphonuclear leukocytes) (PMNs), and monocytes and macrophages (mononuclear leukocytes). These cells engulf organisms (by phagocytosis) without specifically recognising them. Also, they mediate other functions through the secretion of cytokines and the action of enzymes.

The PMNs are usually the first cells at the site of infection and attack invading pathogens whilst producing chemotaxins to attract more polymorphs and mononuclear phagocytes. In addition, PMN products cause changes in host tissues which are vital to the inflammatory process (e.g. vasodilation). Macrophages produce cytokines such as IL-1 and TNF, which cause fever (and enhance the activity of inflammatory cells) and vasodilation, and generally augment the inflammatory process.

Engulfed organisms are enclosed in a **phagosome** which fuses with a **lysosome**. This exposes the organisms to a variety of enzymes and chemicals derived from the lysosomal granules. These processes are adapted to destroy the organisms. However, many have the means to avoid destruction in this manner. Some organisms have extracellular products which inhibit phagocytosis (e.g. the polysaccharide capsules on *Cryptococcus neoformans*, *Streptococcus pneumoniae* and *Haemophilus influenzae*), others resist killing or kill the phagocyte (for example, leucocidin produced by *Staphylococcus* spp. causes the lysosome to release its contents into the cell cytoplasm, which kills the phagocyte).

Phagocytes have been shown to be particularly important in the control of some fungal infections. Normal, healthy individuals rarely suffer from fungal infections, since such organisms are poorly invasive and their spread is limited by the innate immune response until they are eliminated by the adaptive response. Neutrophils may be particularly involved in this control of fungal infections; they are thought to be primarily responsible for preventing the tissue invasion by, and the dissemination of, *Candida* spp.

Eosinophils are particularly important in worm infections in the gut. Antigens released by the infecting worms cross-link Fc receptor-bound IgE on mast cells in the gut mucosa. This induces degranulation of the mast cells, leading to the release of **eosinophil chemotactic factor** (ECF). In addition, T cells in the gut mucosa release **eosinophil stimulation promoter** (ESP). These two factors attract eosinophils to the site and cause their proliferation (ECF and ESP respectively). Eosinophil granules contain a protein — **eosinophil basic protein** — which is particularly toxic to parasites such as *Schistosoma mansoni*. Also, since these cells have Fc receptors, they are able to kill worms by antibody-dependent cellular cytotoxicity (ADCC) (Figure 11.2).

In addition to neutrophils, monocytes/macrophages (mononuclear phagocytes — MNPs) are thought to be important in the clearance of fungi. They may be activated by lymphokines (produced by antigen-stimulated T cells) which enhance their ability to clear the fungi. Also, MNPs have been shown to express surface receptors which bind fungi; however, their role is unclear.

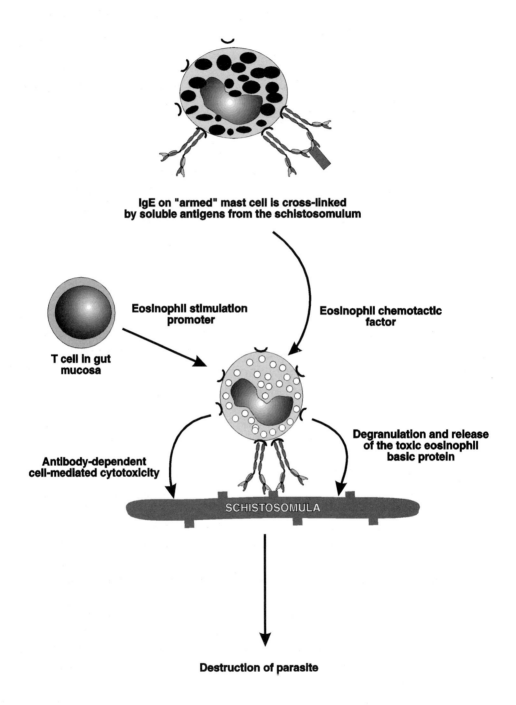

IgE on "armed" mast cell is cross-linked
by soluble antigens from the schistosomulum

Eosinophil stimulation
promoter

Eosinophil chemotactic
factor

T cell in gut
mucosa

Degranulation and release
of the toxic eosinophil
basic protein

Antibody-dependent
cell-mediated cytotoxicity

SCHISTOSOMULA

Destruction of parasite

Figure 11.2   Elimination of parasites by eosinophils

Aspergillus fumigatus attaches to the mannosyl-fucosyl receptors on mouse alveolar macrophages.

Macrophages activated by lymphokines such as interferon-gamma (IFNγ) may kill parasites as a result of increased oxygen metabolism and increased FcR and C3R expression (and therefore more efficient phagocytosis). These cells play a vital role in the control of infections caused by *Trypanosoma cruzi*, *Leishmania* spp., *Plasmodium* spp. and *Schistosoma mansoni*. When parasites are not completely eliminated, granuloma form. Antigens derived from the parasites stimulate T cells to release lymphokines, which in turn stimulate macrophages. These cells release factors which enhance fibrin deposition, resulting in a mesh-work which traps inflammatory cells behind a wall of fibroblasts (**fibrosis**).

Natural Killer Cells

Natural killer (NK) cells are non-adherent, non-phagocytic, large granular lymphocytes. The granules show some similarity to those of MNPs, in that they contain β-glucuronidase. However, they lack peroxidase. The principal characteristics of these cells are that they are able to spontaneously destroy a range of target cells in an MHC-unrestricted manner.

Since many cells are capable of performing NK cell-like activity, particularly after in vitro culture, NK cells are defined as those cells capable of lysing a range of target cells in an MHC-unrestricted manner and expressing a particular range of surface antigens (Table 11.1).

NK cells are produced in the bone marrow, enter the circulation and localise in the tissues. They can be triggered within a few minutes of encountering a target cell but can be activated by cytokines to exhibit even greater activity against a wider range of target cells. However, NK cells do not develop into memory cells or exhibit a secondary response.

Although typically thought to be involved in tissue surveillance and eliminating certain tumours, NK cells are also capable of killing some virally infected targets. These cells may be important in controlling or eliminating viruses even before they replicate and before the development of specific Tc cells.

It has been proposed that NK cells may express antigen receptors which, whilst structurally and functionally distinct from the T cell receptor (TCR), may be clonally distributed. Since T cells (which can perform both MHC-restricted and non-MHC-restricted cytolysis) and NK cells show a number of similarities,

Table 11.1   Surface antigens expressed by NK cells

Marker	Distribution	Function
CD56	NK cells only	Function unknown. Thought to be NK cell specific but some cells do not express it
CD2	T cells and NK cells	Sheep erythrocyte receptor; receptor for LFA1
CD8	Some T cells and NK cells	30–80% human NK cells have CD8 which recognises MHC Class I products
CD11a/CD18 CD11b/CD18	Many leukocytes	LFA1 — the leukocyte functional antigen CR3
CD16	Neutrophils; macrophages	FcγRIII. In NK cells it is capable of mediating ADCC

the signalling pathways leading to T cell activation may be relevant to NK cell activation.

It is common for NK cells to accumulate at the site of an infection. Indeed, viruses stimulate the production of interferon, which enhances NK cell activity, causing them to kill several targets one after the other and to do so more rapidly.

A role for NK cells in recovery from infection has been shown for a number of viruses, including human cytomegalovirus, Epstein–Barr virus, influenza virus, and paramyxoviruses such as mumps, measles and Sendai viruses.

NK cells may also play a role in the destruction of pathogenic fungi. Studies have shown that they may lyse *Cryptococcus neoformans* in a similar way to that in which they cause the destruction of tumour cells, except that attachment occurs more slowly (probably due to the formation of many, small microvilli at the site of attachment) and killing takes longer. By contrast, NK cells are not capable of killing *Candida* spp., indicating that the general role of these cells in controlling or eliminating fungal infections may be limited.

Platelets

In the past, platelets were largely neglected in immunology but it is clear now that they have important roles to play, particularly in parasitic diseases. Platelets from patients infected with *Schistosoma mansoni* are highly cytotoxic to the parasite in vitro. Normal platelets incubated with IgE-rich serum have the same effect, suggesting that the protective activity of platelets is mediated (at least in part) through their ability to bind IgE. Similarly, in vitro studies of trypanosomes have shown that they are rapidly lysed after contact with immune platelets. In addition, the lysis of sensitised *Trypanosoma cruzi* promastigotes is dependent on the presence of the C3b receptor on platelets. These and other experiments have shown that platelets may be protective in parasitic infections through interaction with antibody and complement. However, even in the absence of serum, platelets have been shown to be as effective against *Toxoplasma gondii* as cytotoxic T cells.

THE SPECIFIC IMMUNE RESPONSE

In the same way that humoral and cell-mediated responses are now known to be closely interdependent, the distinction between specific and non-specific immune response to infection has become hard to define. For example, NK cells and macrophages play a role in innate immunity but they may be activated by lymphokines produced as a result of a specific immune response. Also, Fc-receptor-bearing phagocytic cells may act in an antigen-specific manner through binding antibody. When coated with specific antibody, virus-infected cells and other pathogens may be killed by ADCC mediated by macrophages and killer cells.

If the inflammatory response is unable to eliminate an invading organism, the stimulus persists long enough to stimulate a specific immune response. The type of response which predominates is largely dependent on the type of organism causing the infection. Often, both T cell and antibody responses are required to completely eliminate an invading pathogen.

Intracellular pathogens and fungi typically require a cell-mediated response for their elimination. This is demonstrated by the fact that such infections are common in patients infected with the **human immunodeficiency virus (HIV)**, an organism which infects and impairs the activity of the main cells involved in cell-mediated immunity (i.e. CD4+ T cells and macrophages). Although fungal infections are usually eliminated by cell-mediated immunity alone, some require more than this. For example, whilst chronic mucocandidiasis may be cured by effective cell-mediated immunity, recovery from systemic infection with *Candida* spp. requires the activity of granulocytes, cytokines from NK cells and others, complement and possibly humoral immunity. Thus, control of certain fungal infections requires the combined activity of the innate and specific immune responses.

In general, the immune response seems less well equipped to eliminate parasitic infections such as malaria, schistosomiasis and leishmaniasis, which present a major health problem, particularly in the developing world. Over a long period of time, parasites have adapted such that, in general, infection tends to be chronic. As might be expected, cell-mediated immunity is usually more effective against intracellular parasites, whilst antibody tends to play a major role in the elimination of extracellular stages. However, due to the complex developmental cycles of many parasites, a particular immunological mechanism may be more or less effective against a particular stage of a parasite's life cycle.

The Role of Antibody in Immunity to Infection

Antibody is particularly important in controlling disease caused by extracellular organisms. However, the methods of control exhibited by the different classes of antibody differ, depending largely on the type of organism involved and its route of infection. Examples of the roles played by antibodies in immunity to infection are described below and summarised in Figure 11.3.

Opsonisation

Specific antibodies bound to their target organisms may also bind to receptors on phagocytic cells (Fc receptors) but via their Fc portion rather than by the antigen-specific part (the F(ab)$_2$ fragment). This opsonisation increases the phagocytic efficiency of the cells, allowing the organism to be cleared more effectively. In addition, if the antibodies specifically bind flagellar antigens on certain bacteria (e.g. *Salmonella typhi*), they play a secondary role in that they immobilise the organism, thus making it more easy to capture.

Complement Activation

Although antibodies alone may opsonise micro-organisms, complement activation increases phagocytosis and killing still further. In addition, activation of the membrane attack complex (MAC) (C5–C9) results in direct lysis of micro-organisms. However, the type of organism may dictate how efficient the MAC may be. Parasites may be directly damaged due to the activation of complement by antibody bound to the organism. However, bacteria show variability in their susceptibility to lysis. Gram-negative organisms are more easily lysed than Gram-positive organisms. In addition, although the presence of a capsule is considered to protect micro-organisms from immune attack, encapsulated organisms may be lysed by the MAC, provided that the antibodies involved in activation of the complement pathway are directed against the capsular polysaccharides (e.g. *Neisseria meningitidis*).

 The type of antibody involved may influence the role of complement in bacteriolysis. For example, IgM can only mediate killing of Gram-negative bacteria in the presence of complement.

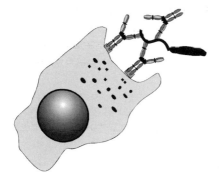

Antibody opsonises the bacterium enhancing phagocytosis

Antibody to flagella antigens prevents motility and increases the efficiency of phagocytosis

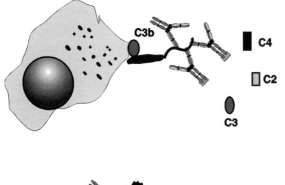

Antibody attached to specific antigen activates the classical complement pathway and kills the micro-organism

Complement also acts as an opsonin and enhances phagocytosis

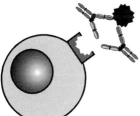

Antibody to viruses, bacteria or parasites may prevent infection by inhibiting cellular attachment

Virus-neutralising antibodies may inhibit virus-cell interaction, prevent endocytosis or prevent its uncoating inside the endosome

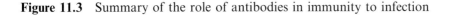

Figure 11.3   Summary of the role of antibodies in immunity to infection

Inhibition of Adherence

Before an organism can cause infection, it has to become attached by binding to a receptor on the cell surface. In bacteria this is often achieved through pili or fimbriae. Antibodies to these organelles may directly inhibit attachment by blocking binding to the receptor on the cell or may sterically hinder such binding.

Similarly, antibodies may inhibit the attachment of viruses to their receptors on their target cells. As with bacteria, this inhibition may be direct, due to stearic hindrance, or may be due to an allosteric effect.

Also, as with bacteria and viruses, antibody may neutralise infection by parasites by preventing attachment to specific cellular receptors (e.g.

Plasmodium spp.). In some infections, antibody is effective in preventing re-invasion of cells by blood-borne parasites (e.g. *Plasmodium falciparum*).

Toxin Neutralisation

Antibodies which bind **exotoxins** secreted by bacteria may neutralise their effect either by preventing their attachment to cellular receptors (e.g. the binding of cholera toxin to the ganglioside GM1) or by enhancing their clearance from the body (through cells with Fc receptors). Immunisation against tetanus works by inducing antibodies which react with the toxin; the latter causes the damage associated with infection.

Virus Neutralisation

Virus neutralisation is a complex process which varies depending upon the type of virus, the target cell and the class of antibody. Since antibodies play an important part in limiting the infectivity of a virus, vaccine performance is often assessed by measuring the level of circulating, neutralising antibodies. Virus-neutralising antibodies may (as described for toxin neutralisation) inhibit virus–cell interaction, prevent endocytosis of the virus or prevent its uncoating inside the endosome. Neutralisation of enveloped viruses may be more effective in the presence of complement.

Inhibition of Microbial Enzyme Activity

Some micro-organisms secrete enzymes (or express them on their surface) which aid in infection (e.g. neuraminidase produced by influenza virus). Antibodies to these enzymes inhibit enzyme function and limit infection.

Inhibition of Microbial Growth

The growth of some prokaryotes may be inhibited by organism-specific antibodies (e.g. *Mycoplasma* spp.).

T Cell-mediated Immunity

Although T cells play a central and critical role in the generation of the immune response to invading micro-organisms, their role is predominantly one of aiding and abetting other cells, rather than directly destroying the organisms themselves. Viruses are the major exception to this rule, since cytotoxic T cells (Tc) are the major form of host defence against established viral infections.

Immune T cells are capable of secreting lymphokines (e.g. IFNγ) which augment the activity of a range of cells, including NK cells and macrophages, which are vital to recovery from infections with viruses such as Herpes simplex. A possible direct role for T cells in antibacterial defence has been suggested by recent studies showing specific lysis of *Listeria monocytogenes*-infected macrophages by sensitised T lymphocytes.

> The role of T cells in fungal infection has been most extensively studied using *Histoplasma capsulatum* in mice. Animals treated with an antibody to remove T helper cells could not eliminate the fungus very efficiently. However, mice given T helper cells from genetically identical (syngeneic) mice resistant to *H. capsulatum* were able to clear the infection, whilst those given normal Th or Ts/c cells from resistant mice did not.

In parasitic infections, Tc cells do not appear to play a vital role in recovery from infections but other T cells are important in prolonging survival of the host, probably by affecting the proliferation of the parasite. Generally, the role of T cells in parasitic infections is to secrete cytokines in response to released antigens. These cytokines increase the activity of eosinophils, mast cells, macrophages and B cells. However, in some parasitic infections (e.g. *Trypanosoma cruzi*) patients with Tc cell activity present with more severe symptoms.

In worm infections, T cells can help to remove the organisms by producing factors which cause goblet cells to secrete more mucus.

Studies of experimental bacterial and parasitic infections have demonstrated differential T cell responses which are dependent on the type of organism eliciting the response. These responses are characterised generally as either Th1 or Th2. In a Th1 response, IL-2, IFNγ and TNF are produced. These are associated with macrophage activation (resulting in enhanced activity against intracellular pathogens and parasites) and stimulation of Tc activity. By contrast, a Th2 response is associated with the secretion of IL-4 and IL-5, which is instrumental in switching B cell immunoglobulin production to IgE and in promoting eosinophil activation, events which are vital to recovery from nematode worm infection. Thus, the production of particular cytokines by T cells may be associated with the activation of different elements of the immune system, the type of response elicited being dependent upon the nature of the infecting organism.

In viral infections, cytokines control antibody responses and influence the early (NK cell activation) and late protective responses (Tc cell activation and proliferation). Since viruses replicate within host cells and virus proteins are expressed in the cell cytoplasm, they present a different challenge to the host immune system than extracellular micro-organisms. Viral antigens are likely to be presented in the context of MHC Class I antigens initially and only later by Class II antigens after viral antigens have been produced and taken up from outside host cells. This results in an initial preferential stimulation of CD8+ T cells.

CYTOTOXIC T CELL ACTIVITY

Once activated, Th1 cells produce cytokines which favour the differentiation of cytotoxic effector and memory cells. These usually express the CD8 antigen but a few may express CD4. In order to express their cytolytic activity, the cytotoxic T cells must bind to their target cells (those which are to be lysed); a process which is temperature, energy and magnesium ion dependent and requires an intact cytoskeleton in the effector T cells. In addition, it has been shown that a stable union between the effector and target cells is dependent upon a number of factors (Table 11.2).

Whilst cytotoxic T cells usually recognise specific processed antigens (which may be foreign or altered self-molecules) in association with MHC molecules on the surface of infected or transformed cells, some bind their target cells via antibodies (which are bound to specific antigens on the target cells) or lectins (compounds which bind sugar residues on cell surface molecules). However, regardless of the means by which effectors and targets become bound, the

---

The complexity of the adhesion process is also reflected structurally. Studies of effector–target cell conjugates by transmission electron microscopy (TEM) revealed extensive folding of the plasma membrane at the site of contact. In this area, the cytoplasm of the Tcs contained a network of fibrillar material but lacked cytoplasmic organelles such as ribosomes and granules. It has been proposed that after the initial period of conjugation, the lytic granules move back into the cytoplasmic projections, allowing them to come into contact with that part of the Tc plasma membrane involved in target cell binding. Thereafter, the granules fuse with the membrane, releasing their lytic contents (such as perforin) into the junctional area between the effector and target cells. Once a lytic signal has been delivered, most Tcs can dissociate from the target cell and attach to further targets at least twice before needing to be reactivated.

---

ultimate outcome of the union is highly variable. The cause of this variability is unknown, but appears to be dependent upon the effector/target cell ratio and the nature of the target cell. Thus, although the attachment between effector and target cells may be brief (the process follows first-order kinetics with a half-life of 1.4 min), the length of time required for cytolysis may vary from

Table 11.2 Parameters affecting the stability of the union between effector and target cells

The union involves contact over a large area of both cells' membranes

Interaction between the TCR–CD8 (or CD4) and processed antigen presented by MHC Class I molecules (or Class II) is required

A 'zipping-up' process involving a group of cell surface antigens called adhesion molecules stabilises the union (e.g. CD2, CD28, CD43, and leukocyte function antigen (LFA)-1 on the effector T cell and B7, CD22, ICAM-1 or ICAM-2 and LFA-3 on the target cell). Some of these molecules also provide co-stimulatory signals for T cell activation (e.g. CD2, CD4, CD8, CD28 and LFA-1)

5 minutes to 24 hours, and, even at high effector/target cell ratios, may be only partial.

Cytolytic Mechanisms

Having been stimulated by cytokines produced by Th1 cells, and having recognised and bound the target cell, the Tc effector cells must induce the lysis of the target cell. Experimental evidence suggests that several different mechanisms of cytolysis may occur (Table 11.3).

After conjugation with a target cell, the Tc delivers its 'lethal hit', an event which requires continued interaction between the TCR–CD3 complex and processed antigen associated with autologous MHC molecules on the target cell (Figure 11.4). The signals or molecules which cause cytolysis are only delivered in the region where the effector and target cells are in close contact, and only the target cell is affected. Once the 'lethal hit' has been delivered, the target cell

Table 11.3 Mechanisms involved in T cell-mediated cytolysis

Mechanisms of cytolysis

Pore formation in the target cell membrane caused by molecules secreted by the effector cells, e.g. perforin and granzymes. This leads to osmotic imbalance, leakage of cytoplasmic components and ultimate cytolysis

Programmed death or apoptosis of the target cell caused by initiation of intracellular signals leading to apoptosis caused by the engagement of certain cell surface receptors, e.g. Fas

Initiation of intracellular signals which lead to cell death caused by certain cytokines, e.g. TNF and IFNγ, upon engagement of their specific cellular receptors

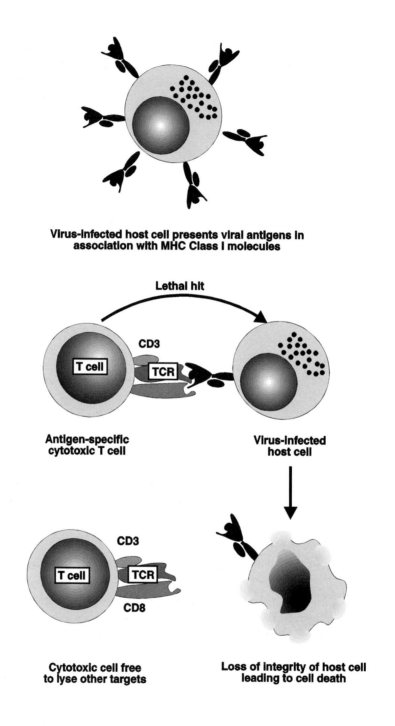

Figure 11.4   Mechanisms of action of cytotoxic T cells

undergoes a number of changes which do not require the further presence of the effector cell.

Complement-like lesions have been seen in target cells lysed by effector lymphocytes thought to be caused by polymerised perforin monomers inserted in the cell membrane. Despite structural similarities between perforin and C9, these molecules have distinct modes of action. Perforin does not require a receptor protein, binding to phosphorylcholine residues on the cell membrane, a process which is calcium-dependent. It can lyse a range of targets, including most nucleated cells, erythrocytes and even lipid vesicles. Perforin monomers bind to the target cell and, after inserting in the plasma membrane, undergo aggregation to form a **hydrophilic channel**, their hydrophobic residues interacting with the acyl chains of membrane phospholipids. This pore leads to osmotic imbalance in the target cell and loss of cytoplasmic contents leading to cytolysis (Figure 11.5).

GRANZYMES

These are a series of enzymes found in the cytoplasmic granules of cytotoxic T cells and NK cells. These granules (which are particularly evident in the early stages of immune activation by certain organisms) contain perforin (a 65–70-kDa glycoprotein which, under certain conditions, shows antigenic similarity to the complement components C6–C9), hydrolytic lysosomal enzymes, several distinct serine proteases and proteoglycans. Although these enzymes are released upon effector–target cell union, convincing evidence that they play an essential role in the lytic process has not been found. However, there is some evidence to suggest that they may act in synergy with perforin to induce lysis.

The initial consequence of the lethal hit from the effector cell is the fragmentation of DNA and blebbing of the target cell membrane. This is typical of cytotoxic T and NK cell-induced **apoptosis**. Typically, the DNA fragments into numerous lengths, each about 180 base pairs long; this is probably caused by cleavage at exposed, intranucleosomal linker regions. This is followed by damage to the target cell's membrane which allows the release of cytoplasmic material and results in the characteristic cell shrinkage and ultimate fragmentation. Apoptosis which occurs as a result of cytotoxic T cell activity is distinct from classical apoptosis, since, usually, the synthesis of relevant molecules by the target is not required. Also, unlike classical apoptosis, in which DNA fragmentation may require hours or days, that induced by cytotoxic T cells is detectable within minutes of effector–target cell interaction.

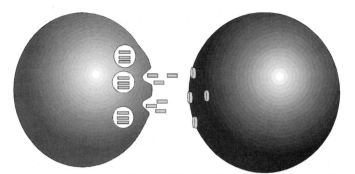

Perforin monomers polymerise and bind to phosphorylcholine residues on the cell membrane

The hydrophilic pore formed results in loss of osmotic balance and cell death

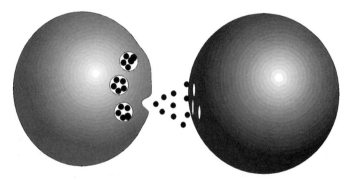

Granzymes are serine esterases found in the cytoplasmic granules of cytotoxic T cells and NK cells

Granzymes may act in synergy with perforin to cause target cell lysis

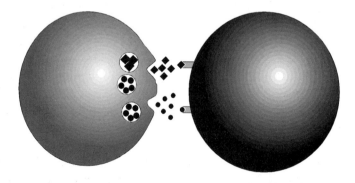

Tumour necrosis factor may cause lysis of target cells by binding to specific receptors on the cell surface

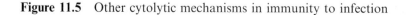

Figure 11.5   Other cytolytic mechanisms in immunity to infection

APOPTOSIS AND NECROSIS

These are two forms of cell death which are quite distinct. During necrosis, the integrity of the cell membrane is destroyed, leading to osmotic imbalance and cell lysis. By contrast, apoptosis is characterised by condensation of nuclear chromatin, ballooning of discrete areas of the cell membrane and fragmentation of the DNA. This causes the cell to shrink and eventually to fragment into membrane-bound apoptotic bodies.

The initiation of apoptosis is dependent upon the appropriate signal being delivered to the target cell nucleus. However, the form of this signal has not been substantiated. The surface antigens APO-1 (on human cells) and Fas (on murine cells) have been shown to be involved in the initiation of apoptosis. Both are anchored in the cytoplasm and are structurally related to the receptor for tumour necrosis factor-alpha.

Cytokines in Immunity to Infection

Apart from cytotoxic effector function, T cells play another important regulatory role in immunity to infection, through the production of cytokines. These affect the activity of a wide range of cells, enhancing the function of some, and inhibiting that of others. In particular, lymphokines activate macrophages, cells which play a vital role in host defence against many bacteria, fungi and parasites.

As described earlier, many extracellular bacteria are most effectively controlled by specific antibody production. The latter requires the activation of specific T cells which produce cytokines to promote the proliferation and differentiation of B cells and the switching of antibody class. We have previously discussed the effect of different cytokines on the proliferation of Th1 and Th2 subsets, and there is clear evidence that recovery from certain infections is dependent upon the predominance of one of these subsets and the cytokines it produces, e.g. trypanosomiasis and Th2 cells.

Intracellular infections are principally controlled by Th1 responses. Products from bacteria and/or parasites stimulate IL-12 production (principally from macrophages) and, thus, early interactions between pathogens and macrophages stimulate the production of IL-12, which initiates a Th1 response. In vivo, IL-12 induces IFNγ production, enhances NK cell activation and promotes protective responses.

The immune response to viral infections may be divided into separate stages, each associated with a particular pattern of cytokine secretion. In the first stage, IFNα/β production causes the activation of NK cells. This may be accompanied by IFNγ and/or IL-12 production. The latter has potent immunoregulatory functions, which include augmentation of the activity of cytotoxic T and NK cells and enhancing the production of IFNγ, which has been shown to enhance Th1 responses whilst inhibiting Th2 responses. In addition, IL-12 has been reported to stimulate similar responses but in an IFNγ-independent fashion.

The replication of viruses inside cells results in the production of a specialised cellular protein, interferon, which acts to limit the infection. Although most viruses stimulate interferon production, the amount produced depends on the virus. DNA viruses are poorer stimulators of interferon than RNA viruses, which include the paramyxoviruses (e.g. Sendai virus), which are the best. After production, interferon diffuses away from the site of infection, inducing an antiviral state in neighbouring cells and preventing the synthesis of viral nucleic acids. These effects collectively inhibit growth and spread of the virus.

Interferon production is one of the earliest host responses to viral infection, and commences within the first 24 hours after invasion. Different types of interferon are produced, depending upon the site of infection and the cells affected. If fibroblasts are among the infected cells, IFNβ is produced. If the site of infection is populated by leukocytes or if the virus spreads to the blood or lymphoid tissue, IFNα is produced. Finally, if T lymphocytes are activated by antigen at the site of infection, IFNγ is also produced. The combined action of these three interferons slows the infection down, with IFNα and IFNβ exerting direct antiviral effects and IFNγ mainly enhancing the immune response (it activates macrophages, augments the activity of NK and Tc cells and increases the expression of MHC molecules on many cells).

Interferon is only effective for a short time and hence plays a major role in acute, short-term infections such as the common cold and influenza. It has no effect on viral multiplication in cells that are already infected.

Following the initial response to virus infection, T cells are activated. This results in the expansion of CD8 + T cells and the production of antigen-specific, Class I-restricted, Tc cells. The cytokines produced during this stage of the response include IL-2, IFNγ, IL-4 and/or IL-10, as well as biologically active transforming growth factor-beta (TGFβ). The role of these cytokines in the generation of active Tc cells is unclear, since studies using IFNγ- and IL-2-deficient mice indicate that these factors are not essential in this process. At this stage of the infection, it is interesting to note that NK cell activity is inhibited but B cells are stimulated. The latter appear to be vital, since in the final stages of the immune response to viral infection, although resolution of infection

Table 11.4 Characteristics of IFNα and IFNβ

Characteristic	Type	Description
Types of interferon		Human interferons comprise: IFNαI (19.2–19.7 kDa), IFNαII (20.1 kDa), IFNβ (20 kDa) and IFNγ Murine interferons comprise: IFNα (19.1 kDa), IFNβ (19.7 kDa) and IFNγ
Major cellular sources	IFNα IFNβ	Lymphocytes, monocytes and macrophages Fibroblasts and some epithelial cells
Effects	IFNα IFNβ	Confers resistance to viruses on target cells, inhibits cell proliferation and regulates expression of MHC Class I antigens Related to IFNα; shares the same receptor and has very similar biological activities
Cross-reactivity	IFNα IFNβ	IFNα shows about 40% homology between humans and mice and there is some species restriction, depending on the particular molecule IFNβ shows about 48% homology in humans and mice; there is **no** cross-species reactivity

Table 11.5 Characteristics of the transforming growth factors

Characteristic		Description
Molecular mass	β	44.3 kDa (human TGFβ1); 47.8 kDa (human TGFβ2); 47.3 kDa (human TGFβ3)
Major cellular sources	β	Platelets contain TGFβ1 and TGFβ2. Most nucleated cell types and many tumours express TGFβ1, TGFβ2 and TGFβ3, or combinations thereof
Effects	β	Involved in tissue remodelling, wound repair, development and haematopoiesis. Inhibits cell growth. Switch factor for IgA
Cross-reactivity	β	TGFβ species show greater than 98% homology in humans and mice

appears to be dependent on Tc cell activity, termination of the immune response is related to antigen clearance, which is mediated by antibody.

> The family of transforming growth factors known as beta are a group of proteins which mediate diverse effects on a variety of cells, such that TGFβ can be either immunosuppressive or immunoenhancing, depending on the cell type involved. TGFβ inhibits the activation of macrophages by IFNγ and prevents the synthesis of reactive oxygen and nitrogen metabolites. Thus, the local production of this cytokine during intracellular infections, e.g. with bacteria or parasites, may be pathogenetic.
>
> In addition, TGFβ inhibits IL-2-dependent cytotoxic T lymphocyte responses but not by interfering with the binding of IL-2 to its receptor.

LEARNING OUTCOMES

Having studied this chapter, you should now appreciate that the body must combat a wide range of infectious agents, each with different characteristics. It achieves this by having a complex network of interdependent defence mechanisms which are selectively activated according to the type of infectious agent involved and the stage of infection. You should now study some specific examples of infection and the elements of the immune system involved in their resolution. You will discover that much of the experimentation has been performed in animals such as mice, and you must remember that the observations may be very different to those in human models. The shortcomings involved in the extrapolation of observations made in animals to humans may be considerable, but since it is often not possible to get pertinent observations from appropriate human tissue, animal studies provide a useful insight into what may be occurring in humans.

Chapter 12

The Immunopathology of Infection

LEARNING OBJECTIVES

We have already looked at the ways in which the immune system tries to prevent infection by a variety of micro-organisms. In many cases, the immune response itself may contribute to the clinical signs and symptoms of the disease caused by a pathogen. Indeed, in a few cases, the immune response may be solely responsible for the clinical disease. Also, the host immune response may help, or even increase, infection in some cases, e.g. the antibody-mediated enhancement of dengue virus infection by Fc-bearing cells such as macrophages. Lastly, some pathogens, particularly viruses, may injure the immune system itself, producing transient or even long-standing immunosuppression. Infection with human immunodeficiency virus (HIV) is the most important example of this type of host–parasite interaction. This chapter is designed to examine these aspects of immunity to infection.

IMMUNOPATHOLOGY

Indirect Damage via the Immune Response

When an immune response occurs, there is, invariably, a certain amount of **inflammation**, cellular infiltration and tissue damage. Such changes caused by the immune response are classed as **immunopathological**. They may be mild and play little or no part in the pathogenesis of disease, or they may be extremely severe, resulting in serious disease or death.

In all infections there is some immunological activity and thus it may be expected that it will contribute to the pathological changes associated with the infection. A typical example of such immunopathology is that which occurs during infection with *Mycobacterium tuberculosis*, where a strong, persistent cell-mediated immune response develops. A typical consequence of infection is tubercle formation, the latter consisting of a central zone (containing bacilli, large mononuclear and giant cells), often with some necrosis, and an outer covering of fibroblasts and lymphocytes. Mononuclear infiltrations, giant cells and granulomatous lesions are characteristic pathological features of tuberculosis. When macrophages are killed by intracellular mycobacteria, the lysosomal enzymes and other materials released from the degenerating cell contribute to the chronic inflammation. Other examples of immunopathological features include the lymph node swelling seen in glandular fever, and the gross enlargement of the spleen caused by chronic malaria and other infections.

The occurrence of pathological changes in some infectious diseases varies from individual to individual. For example, *Chlamydia trachomatis* (which is a major cause of infection in the eyes and genital tract in humans) does not cause pathological changes in most people. However, in some individuals, severe disease develops, leading to blindness and infertility.

Pathology due to the Innate Immune Response

In many instances, the non-specific immune response to an invading pathogen (i.e. the inflammatory response) may be damaging to the host. The release of inflammatory mediators results in pain, swelling and redness of the affected tissues. In addition, enzymes and other factors secreted by polymorphonuclear leukocytes and macrophages may produce permanent tissue damage, which may occasionally lead to loss of function of the affected part. Generally, inflammation is a major cause of the signs and symptoms of disease.

Tissue damage leads (to a greater or lesser extent) to **cellular necrosis** and the release of inflammatory materials. In addition, bacteria themselves may release factors which stimulate inflammation and viruses may induce the release of inflammatory mediators from host cells. Thus, inflammation may be either

---

An example of an organism which releases factors which cause tissue damage and thus stimulate an inflammatory response is *Helicobacter pylori*, the causative agent of human gastritis. This organism excretes urease, which catalyses the hydrolysis of urea to yield ammonia and carbon dioxide. Urease undoubtedly plays a central role in *H. pylori* pathogenesis. Hydrolysis of urea with generation of ammonia may enable survival of this acid-sensitive organism in the gastric mucosa. Ammonia generated by urea hydrolysis may also produce severe cytotoxic effects within the gastric epithelium. Also, the enzyme elicits a strong immune response during acute infection, suggesting that this antigen is readily available to the immune system.

---

a direct or indirect consequence of microbial infection. However, whatever the origin of the stimulus, the resulting inflammatory response may account for the majority of detrimental changes in the tissues. Thus, many pathological changes may be considered to be side-effects of the immune response to infection.

In many diseases, both direct (microbial) and indirect (inflammatory) types of tissue damage make a contribution to the pathology. However, in any particular infection, one or the other phenomenon may predominate. Abscesses caused by *Staphylococcus* spp. result from the effect of inflammatory materials produced by the bacteria and lysosomal enzymes released by polymorpho-nuclear leukocytes which have been killed by the micro-organisms. Similarly, virulent streptococci produce toxins that damage phagocytes. In addition, substances on the surface of these organisms prevent phagocytosis, thus enhancing the persistence of the organisms. However, once specific antibody is produced, most streptococci are phagocytosed and killed and the infection is terminated. Group A streptococci still pose a problem for the immune system, even after they have been killed. The peptidoglycan component of the streptococcal cell wall is resistant to digestion by lysosomal enzymes, and macrophages choked with indigestible cell wall tend to accumulate at sites of infection. Lysosomal enzymes and other substances leak from these cells which locally cause destruction of collagen and connective tissue. The macrophages eventually die or form giant cells, which may result in the formation of granulomas. Thus, the indigestible streptococcal material may cause chronic inflammatory lesions.

Phagocytes also have difficulty digesting other organisms, e.g. *Listeria* spp., *Shigella* spp., *Candida albicans* and *Mycobacterium* spp. However, the relevance of this to the pathogenesis of the resulting disease is, in many instances, unclear.

Factors Affecting or Causing Pathology via the Innate Immune Response

Endotoxin

Bacterial cell walls, or, more accurately, their components, present other problems to the host's immune system than just being indigestible. **Endotoxins**, which form part of the outer layer of the bacterial cell wall, may be released in soluble form during bacterial growth. The word endotoxin generally refers to the complex phospholipid–polysaccharide–protein macromolecules associated with the cell walls of Gram-negative bacteria such as *Salmonella* spp., *Shigella* spp., *Escherichia* spp. and *Neisseria* spp. The **lipopolysaccharide (LPS)** is the important component from a clinical point of view (Figure 12.1). The LPS of Gram-negative bacteria consists of three components, a **core polysaccharide** common to many Gram-negative bacteria, an **O-specific polysaccharide** which confers virulence and serological specificity on the macromolecule, and a **lipid A** component which is mainly responsible for the toxicity of the molecule. LPS is an important **virulence factor** and small changes in the O antigen, involving no

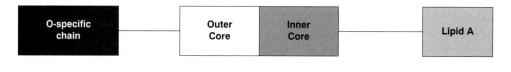

Structure found in Enterobacteriaceae, Pseudomonadaceae.

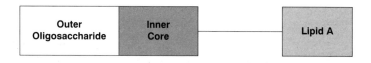

Structure found in *Neisseria meningitidis, Haemophilus influenzae, Bordetella pertussis, Acinetobacter calcoaceticus, Bacteroides fragilis.*

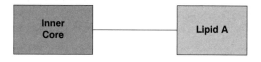

Structure found in *Chlamydia trachomatis, Chlamydia psittaci.*

Figure 12.1   Structure of lipopolysaccharide

more than changes in the sugar sequences in side chains of the molecule, result in major changes in virulence.

Endotoxin-induced Injury

Endotoxin-mediated host injury, which clinically results in the **sepsis syndrome** or **septic shock**, is usually consequent to severe infection by Gram-negative bacteria such as *Meningococcus* spp. In this instance, much of the resulting disease is attributable to the host response to the endotoxin, not to direct injury by the endotoxin itself. LPS causes the release of **vasoactive substances** and activates both the alternative complement pathway and factor XII (Hageman factor of the coagulation cascade). This latter capability sometimes results in the development of disseminated intravascular coagulation. With respect to the pathology associated with the sepsis syndrome, perhaps the most relevant effect of LPS is its ability to stimulate macrophages to release interleukin-1 (IL-1) and tumour necrosis factor (TNF). Endotoxins are also pyogenic; LPS causes the release of IL-1 from macrophages which acts on the hypothalamus to give a rapid elevation of body temperature.

Adhesion Molecules

The pathology of many parasitic diseases is affected by adhesion molecules which are expressed on the surface of cells and promote cell–cell adhesion (Figure 12.2). These molecules may be used by microbes to facilitate attachment and invasion and ultimately (in many cases) to increase tissue damage. For example, the adhesion of parasite-infected erythrocytes to brain endothelium may be a primary event in cerebral malaria in humans and is thought to involve CD36 and thrombospondin. In addition, the adhesion molecule **ICAM-1** has been implicated in malaria, since its expression on vascular endothelium can be upregulated by TNF, and increased levels of this cytokine have been shown to correlate with disease severity.

> The cDNA of CD36 has been expressed in COS cells. When these cells were mixed with red blood cells infected with *Plasmodium falciparum*, they were found to bind to each other, the binding being inhibited by an antibody to CD36.

Heat Shock Proteins

Heat shock proteins are a group of molecules found in both eukaryotes and prokaryotes which exhibit an extremely high level of conservation. This means that the structures of the proteins in humans are extremely similar to those of the equivalent molecules found in simpler forms of life. This degree of conservation would imply that these molecules have an important role in the normal functioning of the organism concerned. Heat shock protein synthesis increases as a result of cellular stress in the form of severe temperature fluctuations, viral infection, oxidative stress and fever, to name but a few. Peptides derived from these proteins are thought to be recognised by the small population of T cells (in humans) which bear an antigen receptor comprised of γ and δ chains (T$\gamma\delta$). Heat shock proteins may be released from damaged bacteria, stimulating T cells; this, because of the highly conserved nature of the

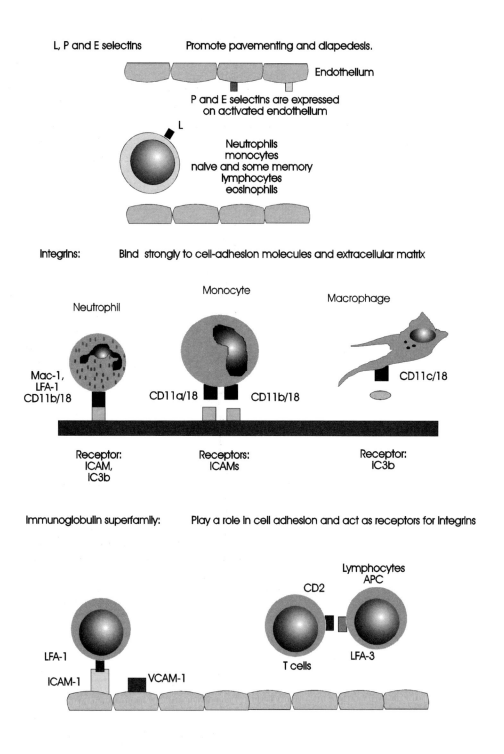

Figure 12.2   Examples of adhesion molecules

proteins, may result in a breakdown of tolerance to self and the development of autoimmune phenomena.

> Infection with *Chlamydia trachomatis* in some individuals leads to the development of severe disease which results in blindness and infertility. A chlamydial protein—HypB—which belongs to the 60-kDa family of heat shock proteins (hsp 60) has been identified as the constituent which stimulates the immune response which causes the severe pathology.

Pathology due to Specific Antibody

There are many examples of host injury which occurs as a result of the **humoral immune response** to a pathogen; some of these are shown in Table 12.1.

The occurrence of **cross-reactive antigens** is quite frequent, and a number of micro-organisms stimulate the production of antibodies which are capable of reacting to host tissue components, giving rise to autoimmune damage. Typical examples of this include chorea and rheumatic fever (Table 12.1).

Table 12.1 Examples of injury caused by pathogen-stimulated antibody

Disease or clinical presentation	Infectious agent	Immune phenomena and pathology
Post-streptococcal glomerulonephritis	*Streptococcus* spp.	Immune complexes containing streptococcal antigens and IgG deposit in the kidney, activating complement and attracting inflammatory cells
Polyarteritis nodosa	Hepatitis B virus	Chronic antigen–antibody complex formation causes activation of complement and signs and symptoms of chronic inflammation
Chorea	*Streptococcus* sp.	Antibodies stimulated by the streptococcal infection react with neurons in the caudate and subthalamic nuclei of the brain
Rheumatic fever	Throat infection with group A *Streptococcus* sp.	Antibodies formed against streptococcal cell walls or membrane components also react with patient's heart muscle or valves, resulting in myocarditis

Several infectious agents are thought to cause the polyclonal activation of B cells which results in the production of antibodies which react with self-antigens. The latter include DNA, immunoglobulin, myofibrils and erythrocytes. Such autoantibodies have been demonstrated in patients infected with trypanosomes, *Mycoplasma pneumoniae* and Epstein–Barr virus. Although it is unclear precisely what contribution these autoantibodies make to the pathology of each of these diseases, their production alone reflects a fundamental disturbance of the patient's normal immunoregulatory system which is a pathological consequence of infection in itself.

In many instances of microbial infection, the resulting pathology is caused by the immune response which may be classified as a **hypersensitivity reaction**. The antibody-mediated destruction of infected cells which results in tissue damage (a classical type II hypersensitivity response) may be the cause of some of the liver necrosis seen in hepatitis B and yellow fever. The haemolysis associated with malaria is caused (in part) in this way. In addition, *Mycoplasma pneumoniae* causes an atypical pneumonia in which antibodies (cold agglutinins) are formed against normal human group O erythrocytes, occasionally resulting in haemolytic anaemia.

When antigen–antibody reactions take place in extravascular tissues, there is inflammation and oedema with infiltration of PMNs (Figure 12.3). If soluble antigen is injected intradermally into an individual with large amounts of circulating IgG antibody, the antigen–antibody reaction takes place in the walls of skin blood vessels and causes an inflammatory response. The extravasating PMNs degenerate and their lysosomal enzymes cause extensive vascular damage. This is known as a classical **Arthus response**. Antigen–antibody reactions in tissues do not usually have such serious implications, and the consequences of an inflammatory response are commonly quite minimal. Indeed, IgA-containing immune complexes are less harmful. Antigens absorbed from the gut combine with locally produced IgA, the resulting complex entering the circulation to be filtered out in the liver and excreted in the bile.

When antigen–antibody reactions take place in the blood, the consequences of the presence of circulating immune complexes are directly related to the size of the immune complexes and the relative proportions of antigen and antibody therein (Figure 12.4). In antibody excess, the antigen becomes coated with antibody and is removed rapidly by cells of the mononuclear phagocyte system which have Fc and complement receptors. At antibody–antigen equivalence, large lattices are formed, their size enabling their rapid clearance. By contrast, antigen is present in large excess; few antibody molecules coat each antigen, thus reducing the likelihood of clearance. These complexes therefore continue to circulate in the blood and may become localised in small blood vessels, e.g. in the glomeruli of the kidneys, the choroid plexuses, the joints and the ciliary body of the eye. It is thought that factors such as local high blood pressure and turbulent flow (glomeruli) or the

Circulating immune complexes formed during severe generalised infections such as Gram-negative septicaemia, meningococcal septicaemia, plague, yellow fever and other haemorrhagic arthropod-borne viruses very infrequently cause a severe condition known as disseminated intravascular coagulation. Enzymes of the coagulation pathway are activated by the immune complexes, leading to histamine release, increased vascular permeability and fibrin deposition in the blood vessels of the kidneys, lungs, adrenals and pituitary. This results in the local formation of numerous blood clots (thromboses) which locally prevent blood flow and cause tissue damage (infarcts). In addition, haemorrhages occur due to the depletion of platelets and a number of factors involved in blood clotting, such as prothrombin and fibrinogen.

filtering function of vessels involved (choroid plexus, ciliary body) may influence the deposition of these small immune complexes. In the glomeruli, they pass through the endothelium and may localise beneath the basement membrane, although the smallest appear to pass through the basement membrane and enter the urine. This may be a normal mechanism for disposing of such complexes.

When an immune response is first generated, immune complexes are formed in antigen excess. However, there is usually only a very brief period before specific antibody levels in the blood rise, resulting in the formation of immune complexes which contain equivalent or higher levels of antibody than antigen. However, in some instances, small immune complexes persist and localise in the kidney glomeruli, where they activate complement and induce an inflammatory response. This results in PMN infiltration, glomerular basement membrane swelling, and albumin and red blood cells in the urine. This **acute glomerulonephritis** may be seen mainly in children as a post-infection complication with *Streptococcus* spp. When the immune system has eliminated the infection, immune complexes are no longer formed, and any pathological changes are usually reversed, leading to complete recovery. However, repeated infection or the persistent deposition of complexes leads to irreversible damage. This happens in certain persistent infections in which microbial antigens are released continuously into the blood but antibody responses are weak or of low affinity. In such cases, immune complexes localise in the glomeruli over a period of weeks, months or even years, and ultimately cause impairment of their filtering function.

Circulating immune complexes may be deposited in other locations in the body and cause classical pathology. For example, immune complexes which localise in the joints lead to joint swelling and inflammation. The **prodromal rashes** seen in some viral infections and in hepatitis B are probably caused by

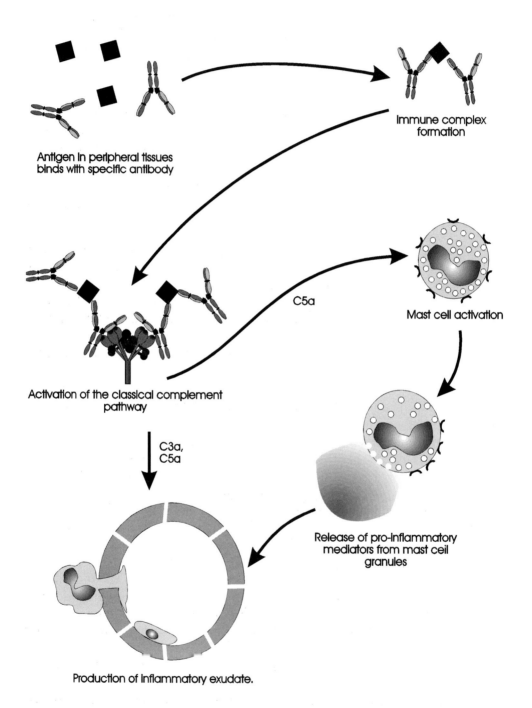

Figure 12.3 Effect of immune complex formation in extravascular tissues

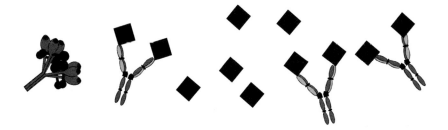

Antigen excess: poor level of opsonisation which makes phagocytosis difficult

Complement cannot bind

Immune complexes persist

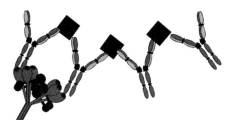

Antibody/antigen equivalence
Complexes easily phagocytosed

Complexes cleared

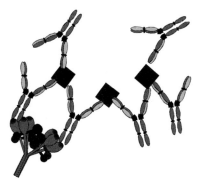

Antibody excess
Complexes easily phagocytosed

Complexes cleared

Figure 12.4   The influence of the structure of immune complexes on their own clearance

immune complexes being deposited in the walls of small blood vessels in the skin. If the vascular changes are more marked (as is seen following streptococcal infections and in patients being treated for leprosy), they give rise to the condition called **erythema nodosum**, in which there are tender, red nodules in the skin with deposits of antigen, antibody and complement in vessel walls.

When immune complexes are formed in the airways, the resulting inflammatory response causes wheezing and respiratory distress, giving rise to the condition known as allergic alveolitis. Repeated inhalation of the antigen concerned leads to chronic, pathological changes which result in fibrosis and respiratory disease, e.g. Farmer's lung caused by the actinomycete *Micromonospora faeni*, found in mouldy hay.

The pathology associated with a number of infectious diseases may be mediated by immune complexes. Indeed, the fever, polyarthritis, skin rashes and kidney damage seen in meningococcal meningitis and gonococcal septicaemia are indicative of immune complex deposition. Also, the oedema and vasculitis of trypanosomiasis and the rashes of secondary syphilis may be a consequence of immune complex formation.

Pathology caused by the Cell-mediated Immune Response

The mere expression of a cell-mediated immune response involves some degree of inflammation, lymphocyte infiltration, macrophage accumulation and activation, and can therefore by itself cause pathological changes. This type of response predominates in the pathogenesis of tuberculosis, with mononuclear cell infiltration, degeneration of parasitised macrophages and the formation of giant cells as central features. In chronic mycobacterial infection, the continuous release of microbial antigens leads to a chronic inflammatory response and the formation of granulomas (Figure 12.5). This particular pathological feature is also associated with a range of other chronic microbial and parasitic diseases, including bacterial (actinomycosis, leprosy and syphilis), chlamydial (lymphogranuloma inguinale) and fungal (coccidiomycosis) infections.

Granuloma formation is associated with antigen persistence and so the glucan of *Candida albicans* (which is more resistant to breakdown in macrophages) is responsible for the chronic inflammatory responses associated with infection, despite mannan being the dominant antigen.

Mononuclear cells also cause pathological changes during a cell-mediated response by lysing host cells. When the latter are infected by a virus, viral antigens are expressed on their surface, providing a target for cell-mediated responses. In this way, cell-mediated immunity may contribute to the pathology of hepatitis B infection and many herpes and pox virus infections. Also, the autoimmune damage associated with Chagas' disease may be due to the adsorption of antigens from *Trypanosoma cruzi* on uninfected host cells, allowing recognition by cytotoxic T cells or destruction by antibody-dependent cellular cytotoxicity.

Chagas' disease is caused by *Trypanosoma cruzi* and is transmitted by blood-sucking insects. The organisms spread throughout the body during the acute infection. Years later, a poorly understood chronic disease appears, involving the heart and the intestinal tract. These organs contain only small numbers of the parasite but show a loss of autonomic ganglion cells. It is thought that the pathology arises as a result of an autoimmune reaction, since a monoclonal antibody to *T. cruzi* has been obtained which cross-reacts with mammalian neurons.

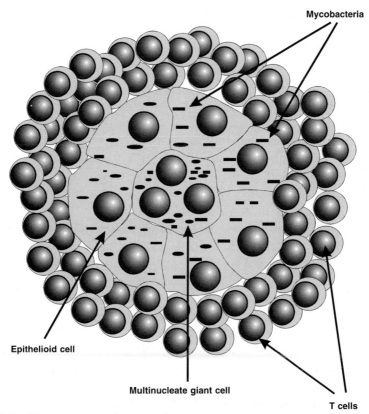

Figure 12.5   The structure of a granuloma

One human virus infection in which a cell-mediated immune response appears to contribute greatly to the pathology of the disease is **measles**. This is evidenced by the fact that children with thymic aplasia suffer a fatal disease if they are infected with measles virus. Individuals with this particular immunodeficiency generally fail to develop antigen-specific T cell responses and cell-mediated immunity but have normal antibody responses. Thus, instead of the limited virus growth and respiratory disease seen in normal children, those with thymic aplasia show uncontrolled virus replication in the lung (despite specific antibody formation), resulting in giant cell pneumonia. Also, the typical measles rash is absent. These studies indicate that the cell-mediated immune response is essential for regulation of virus growth and for the production of the characteristic skin lesions. Other studies have suggested that a similar conclusion can be drawn about the rashes in pox virus infection.

The toxins of *Staphylococcus aureus* and *Streptococcus pyogenes* belong to a family of **exotoxins** which have a profound effect on the immune system. These bacterial **superantigens** promote cell-mediated immunity by stimulating T cell activation and recruitment to local sites of inflammation. The T cell-stimulating activity contributes to the pathogenesis of the respective disease.

Superantigens

Superantigens stimulate both CD4- and C8-positive T cells, as well as a fraction of T cells with antigen receptors which are composed of γ and δ chains (T$\gamma\delta$). Stimulation is caused by cross-linking variable parts of the T cell antigen receptor and non-polymorphic parts of the MHC Class II molecules on antigen-presenting cells (Figure 12.6). For T cells which bear an antigen receptor composed of α and β chains (T$\alpha\beta$), the variable region of the β chain provides the site of attachment for the superantigen.

The T cell activation properties of superantigens have been implicated in a number of diseases where the consequence of this activation is pathogenetic. In allergy, superantigens induce the production of the pro-inflammatory cytokines IL-1 and TNFα, which enhance the expression of **E-selectin**. The complementary molecule for E-selectin is **cutaneous lymphocyte-associated antigen (CLA)**, which is found on T cells invading the skin in allergic individuals; its expression is induced by IL-12, presumably released by Langerhans cells or other antigen-presenting cells upon stimulation with superantigen. Much of this work was performed in vitro, and confirmation in vivo is still awaited.

Evidence that superantigens also influence antibody-mediated allergic responses is largely anecdotal but quite convincing (Table 12.2).

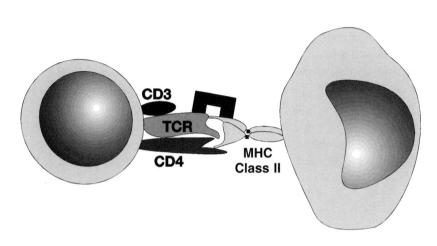

**Superantigen is not processed and binds outside of the cleft
on the MHC Class II molecule**

It also binds outside of the antigen-binding site on the β chain of the TCR

Figure 12.6   Superantigen stimulation of T cells

Table 12.2   Evidence of a role for superantigen in atopic dermatitis

Evidence
Staphylococcus aureus isolated from skin lesions of patients with atopic dermatitis secrete large amounts of superantigen whilst those isolated from non-atopic (allergic) individuals do not
Skin colonisation by *Staph. aureus* can cause severe exacerbation of atopic dermatitis
Anti-*Staph. aureus* superantigen IgE has been found in patients undergoing exacerbation of atopic dermatitis due to *Staph. aureus* colonisation
Peripheral blood basophils 'armed' with anti-*Staph. aureus* superantigen IgE undergo degranulation and release histamine upon challenge in vitro with superantigen

LEARNING OUTCOMES

This chapter was designed to introduce you to the concept that the immune response may be detrimental rather than beneficial and that this may be due to the ability of micro-organisms to adapt and take advantage of our immune systems. You should now have an understanding of precisely how the humoral and cell-mediated immune responses may, during an infection, cause tissue damage and disease. You should also appreciate how such infection can cause pathological changes which result from the breakdown of tolerance and the development of autoimmune reactions. Finally, you have been given examples of pathological changes brought about by hypersensitivity reactions to particular micro-organisms. You should now read the references listed in the Further Reading to give you a fuller understanding of the mechanisms involved in the development of the immunopathology of infectious diseases.

Chapter 13

Tumour Immunology

LEARNING OBJECTIVES

The term **cancer** is used to describe a wide range of disease states involving nearly every type of tissue in the body. Cancer cells lose the functional and phenotypic characteristics of the tissue from which they are derived and are said to have undergone **malignant transformation** and to be **de-differentiated**. As the malignancy progresses, the cancer cells compete with normal ones for both physical space and for nutrients. Some malignancies are capable of breaking up and spreading via the circulatory or lymphatic systems to remote sites of the body. As a result, new foci of malignant cell growth (**metastases**) are established far removed from the original tissue in which the cancer developed. This chapter is designed to introduce you to those characteristics of cancer cells which may allow control by the immune system or which enable the tumour to escape immune surveillance.

THE NATURE OF MALIGNANT DISEASE

Normally, the differentiation and proliferation of cells is largely governed by their stage of development and by the nature of the tissue from which they derive. Organs and tissues have discrete structures and defined histological make-ups, within which the rate of cell death is balanced with the rate of the production of new cells. In some pathological conditions, the production of a particular stimulus may lead to increased cell proliferation such that the number of new cells exceeds that of dying cells. This results in **organ hypertrophy**. When the stimulus is eliminated, cell proliferation decreases and the hypertrophy resolves. By contrast, if a cell undergoes malignant transformation (i.e. it becomes a tumour cell), it is able to replicate without any stimulus. This ability to grow unchecked allows the tumour cells to invade and disrupt local tissues, preventing their normal function and, if untreated, causing death. The poor **prognosis** (expected outcome) of a number of cancers is a direct result of this ability as well as their ability to metastasise and grow in distant organs. Some characteristics of malignant cells are summarised in Table 13.1.

CAUSES OF MALIGNANCY

The transformation of a normal cell into a malignant one can result from a wide range of causes, the nature of which determines whether or not the growth of the tumour may be controlled by the immune system. Transformation may occur spontaneously (as a result of **gene rearrangements** or **random mutations**), or they may be induced by viral, chemical or physical carcinogens (cancer-promoting substances).

Physical Carcinogens

The discovery and subsequent use of X-rays and radioactivity in the late 19th century resulted in the first examples of cancer caused by physical carcinogens. In more recent years, the most convincing evidence of radiation-induced carcinogenesis has come from studies of the survivors of the Hiroshima atomic bomb and the population who lived in the vicinity of the Chernobyl atomic energy plant. These people have presented with increased incidences of a range of tumours, usually several years after the event. Ionising radiation is thought to directly damage DNA, resulting in **mutation**, **abnormal gene rearrangements** and **chromosomal breakage**. However, the long period between exposure and appearance of the tumour suggests that some other genetic event or the activation of a promoter is required for tumour development.

Table 13.1   Common properties of tumour cells

Tumour cells:
fail to respond to signals which normally regulate cell growth and tissue repair
exhibit autonomous (self-directed, independent) growth, i.e. they do not require outside (exogenous) signals
invade normal tissues and, unlike normal cells, their growth is not inhibited by tissue boundaries
metastasise, i.e. they are capable of spreading into distant organs through the lymphatic and blood circulation and there establish new foci of growth
exhibit phenotypic and antigenic differences from non-transformed cells in the same tissue
are monoclonal in origin but heterogeneity may develop at the phenotypic and genetic level as the tumour grows

In recent years, there has been a distinct increase in the incidence of skin cancer, particularly in sunny countries such as Australia. Evidence suggests that this is related to increased exposure to UV light, which may cause the production of carcinogenic **oxygen metabolites** and **pyrimidine dimers**.

Chemical Carcinogens

Tumours induced by chemical carcinogens were initially described in the 18th century when chimney sweeps were observed to have an unusually high incidence of carcinoma of the scrotum. It is believed that tar in the wrinkles of the scrotum was responsible for these tumours, since the **polycyclic aromatic hydrocarbons** in soot and tar have been found to be a major class of carcinogens. Other aromatic hydrocarbons such as the **aromatic amines** have been implicated in malignancy due to the observation of a high frequency of bladder cancer among factory workers using **aniline dyes**.

Viral Carcinogens

Cells transformed by viral genes may be expected to express viral antigens which may be capable of stimulating an immune response. Thus, tumours caused by oncogenic (tumour-causing) viruses may present an opportunity for immunological control or elimination of the tumour.

Oncogenic viruses may contain either DNA or RNA. When a potentially oncogenic virus infects a permissive cell (i.e. one which allows viral replication), infection usually results in cell lysis. However, if a non-permissive cell is infected by the same virus, the viral DNA may integrate into the host cell genome. The resulting **transformation** of the cell may result from viral DNA triggering host genes or from the abnormal splicing of viral mRNA by the host which results in the production of novel transformation-promoting proteins. Although oncogenic DNA viruses have not been isolated from human tumours, the incidence of several viruses has been linked statistically with certain tumours (Table 13.2).

Table 13.2 Some examples of carcinomas and their causative agents

Agent	Outcome
Epstein–Barr virus	Burkitt's lymphoma
Papilloma virus	Cervical cancer
Hepatitis B	Hepatocellular carcinoma
HTLV-1	Lymphocytic leukaemia and lymphoma
Benzene derivatives; nitrogen mustard	Damage DNA
Gamma irradiation	Induces malignancies

Retroviruses contain RNA (rather than DNA) and possess genes which code for the polymerase enzyme—**reverse transcriptase**. This produces a DNA copy of the viral RNA which can be integrated (incorporated) into the host genome. Oncogenic retroviruses were isolated first from chicken tumours and have subsequently been shown to be responsible for a large number of cancers in many different species, e.g. the human T cell leukaemia virus (HTLV). Some cause transformation directly through the presence of **oncogenes** (see below) in their genomes, while others activate the host's genes.

Oncogenes

Several genes have been identified in normal cells which, when activated under appropriate conditions, lead to the malignant transformation of the cell. Some of these cellular oncogenes have been shown to have a role to play in normal growth and development. However, changes which cause the permanently active transcription of these genes are thought to cause the malignant transformation of the cell (Table 13.3).

Oncogenes have been shown to code for membrane receptors, autocrine growth factors and regulators of gene expression. In malignant cells, the products of these genes are increased and thus may make the malignant cells immunologically distinct from the normal cells in the surrounding tissues.

TUMOUR ANTIGENS

Tumours which arise spontaneously, often as a result of exposure to environmental carcinogens, lack distinct dominant antigens, making it difficult to identify tumour-specific immune responses. However, in recent years techniques have been developed which have allowed the expansion of tumour-antigen-specific T and B cells from patients with melanoma, breast cancer, leukaemia, lymphoma and lung cancer; these are present only in extremely low numbers.

Table 13.3   Examples of some events which result in malignant transformation

Event
Mutation of a regulatory gene which may interfere with its activity
Translocation of an oncogene next to an active cellular gene (e.g. in some B cell lymphomas, translocation of an oncogene next to an immunoglobulin variable region gene has been demonstrated), resulting in its inappropriate activation
Insertion of a promoter that enhances the expression of an oncogene

Table 13.4 Mechanisms involved in tumour antigen production

Cause	Explanation
Viral gene transcription	A transforming event may lead to the transcription of integrated retroviral genes and the subsequent expression on the cell surface of viral proteins
Chemical production of aberrant proteins	Chemicals may cause the production of aberrant cellular proteins by interfering at particular stages of their normal production, e.g. during truncation or glycosylation. Degradation of these abnormal compounds may lead to the surface expression of unique antigens
Chemically induced genetic mutation leading to altered molecular structure	Chemicals may cause genetic mutations resulting in the altered structure of cell surface antigens and thus their antigenicity, e.g. major and minor histocompatibility antigens on tumours induced by chemical carcinogens. Some tumour antigens may result from the exposure of antigenic determinants due to mutations which result in the deletion of parts of a molecule, e.g. loss of glycosylation sites in glycolipid antigens
Genetic mutation leading to incorrect assembly of complex molecules	Mutation in one component of a multimeric membrane protein may prevent correct assembly, resulting in the exposure of normally concealed antigenic determinants
Abnormal expression of antigens	Tumour antigens may result from the abnormal expression of fetal or differentiation antigens, e.g. human gastric carcinoma cells express ABO blood group antigens which do not match the self blood type

Tumour antigens may arise by a number of different pathways, some of which are described in Table 13.4.

Transformed cells often express antigens that are seen usually only in utero, e.g. α-fetoprotein and carcinoembryonic antigen. These 'immature antigens' may be indicative of the de-differentiated nature of transformed cells and are often referred to as **tumour-associated antigens**.

Tumour-associated Antigens

Tumour-associated antigens (TAA) are not unique to tumour cells; they may also be found on some normal cells. However, the presence of these antigens may be dependent on the state of differentiation of the normal cells and may differ qualitatively (i.e. they may be expressed together with other markers specific for a particular stage of cell development) or quantitatively (in higher or lower concentration) from that on tumour cells, allowing the use of these antigens to distinguish between the two cell types.

The best characterised human TAAs are the **oncofetal antigens** (carcino-embryonic antigen and α-fetoprotein), which are expressed on the developing embryo (i.e. during embryogenesis) but are absent generally in normal adult tissues.

Carcinoembryonic Antigen

Carcinoembryonic antigen (CEA) is a glycoprotein found on fetal gut cells and on colorectal tumours (tumours affecting the colon and rectum). However, serum levels of CEA are also raised in patients with colitis (itis — inflammation; inflammation of the colon), pancreatitis and pancreatic, lung and breast cancers. Thus, although elevated serum CEA levels may not be indicative of cancer of the colon, measurement of these levels during treatment has been shown to be a prognostic marker for tumour progression and response to treatment.

α-Fetoprotein

α-Fetoprotein is a glycoprotein (70 kDa) expressed mainly by the yolk sac and liver of the fetus. Formerly, it was thought that serum levels decline in the final weeks before birth and, shortly thereafter, completely disappear. Thus, the detection of this antigen in adults with liver cancer was thought to be diagnostic of this condition. However, with the development of highly sensitive assays, it has been demonstrated that low levels of α-fetoprotein may be found in normal

Table 13.5   Other tumour-associated antigens

Antigen	Distribution
CD5	Normally expressed on immature T cells, commonly expressed on malignant B cells found in chronic lymphocytic leukaemia
CALLA or CD10	Expressed minimally on cells such as granulocytes and kidney cells; it is the common acute lymphocytic leukaemia antigen

adult sera, in patients with acute hepatitis and in pregnant women. Thus, α-fetoprotein is not a tumour-specific antigen but a tumour-associated antigen.

Tumour-specific Antigens

Tumour-specific antigens (TSA) are expressed only on tumour cells and are distinct from those on any normal cell. Indeed, these antigens may be unique to a particular patient rather than to a particular tumour. Although the characterisation of certain TSAs is, as yet, incomplete, there is some evidence that they can stimulate a specific immune response.

Common Tumour Antigens

Common tumour markers are found on the membranes of nearly all types of tumour cell. They are a poorly characterised group of **glycolipid antigens** but there is some evidence that they may be a type of **ganglioside**. Evidence suggests that these markers may stimulate innate immunity, leading to the recognition and lysis of the tumour cells by natural killer cells and mononuclear phagocytes.

Tumour-suppressing Genes

Tumour-suppressing genes are found in normal cells and are thought to code for DNA-binding proteins which regulate gene expression and prevent excessive cellular proliferation. However, it is not clear as to precisely how these **anti-oncogenes** prevent malignancy or how malignancy develops when they are functionally defective. It is thought that the combination of a number of different factors results in malignancy. These factors include the loss of tumour-protecting genes and the over-expression of normal or mutated **proto-oncogenes**.

TUMOUR IMMUNOLOGY

The immune system, at least theoretically, has the potential to control the outgrowth of malignant cells. However, the observation that immunodeficient individuals do not show an increased incidence of immunogenic tumours suggests that the regulation of tumour cell growth is more complex. Clearly, the ability of particular tumour cells to stimulate antigen-specific effector mechanisms such as antibody-mediated cellular cytotoxicity and T cell-mediated cytolysis will depend upon their antigenicity. These mechanisms are likely to be most effective against highly immunogenic tumours (e.g. those induced by oncogenic viruses), whilst non-specific effector responses (e.g. NK and LAK cell activity) are likely to be of greater importance with less immunogenic tumours. It is thought that the initial appearance of transformed cells may be controlled by non-specific effector mechanisms and that failure of these to eliminate the malignancy results in the stimulation (at some later stage of development) of tumour-specific immune responses. This is supported by observations of the regression of metastatic lesions after the removal of primary tumours and of the spontaneous regression of tumours.

Although theoretically we might expect the immune system to control tumour cell growth, clinical studies show that many tumours do not provoke an immune response or, if they do so, the response is clearly ineffective. This may be because many tumours appear to possess the ability to evade or overcome the potentially lethal immune response.

Effector Mechanisms Involved in Tumour Immunology

T Cells

In tumour-bearing patients, the T cell response may cause direct killing of tumour cells and activate other components of the immune system capable of exerting control over tumour cell growth. Immunity to tumours involves both CD4+, Class II-restricted, and Class I-restricted, CD8+, T cells. The former are largely Th cells that secrete lymphokines which activate other effector cells (e.g. cytotoxic T and B cells) and enhance inflammatory responses. The CD8+ T cells are mostly cytotoxic, causing direct lysis of tumour cells. However, these cells are also capable of producing lymphokines.

Since tumour cells generally express Class I rather than Class II MHC molecules, Th cells are unable to recognise the transformed cells themselves and must rely on antigen-presenting cells to present tumour-derived antigens. Once stimulated by antigen, Th cells secrete lymphokines that activate Tc cells, macrophages, NK cells (Th1 cells) and B cells (Th2 cells). These cells also produce tumour necrosis factor (TNF), which may be directly lytic to tumour cells.

In contrast to Th cells, the cytotoxic T cells are able to directly recognise and kill tumour targets by disrupting the membrane and nucleus of the latter.

B Cells and Antibody-dependent Killing

Occasionally it has proven possible to identify tumour-reactive antibodies in the serum of patients. This suggests that antibodies may play a role in the immune response to tumours. This is also supported by the fact that B cell lines producing antibodies to TAAs have been derived from the draining lymph nodes of human tumours. Such tumour-reactive B cells may also play an important role in the processing and presentation of tumour antigens to Th cells.

Table 13.6   Characteristics of the tumour necrosis factors

Characteristic	Description
Molecular mass	TNFα has cysteine residues which form intrachain disulphide bonds. It has a molecular mass of 17.4 kDa in humans, 17.3 kDa in mice. TNFβ is a glycosylated molecule with a molecular mass of 18.7 kDa in humans and 18.6 kDa in mice. The genes for both are on chromosome 6 in humans and 17 in mice
Major cellular sources	TNFα is produced by activated monocytes and macrophages, by B cells, T cells and fibroblasts, whilst TNFβ is produced by activated T cells
Effects	TNFα regulates the growth and differentiation of many cell types. It is selectively cytotoxic for many transformed cells and mediates many of its effects in concert with other cytokines. Expressed as a type II membrane protein, TNFβ has 35% homology with TNFα and binds to the same receptor. It is involved in inflammation and immune function and is cytotoxic or cytostatic for some tumours in vitro, and causes haemorrhagic necrosis of certain tumours in vivo. It induces gene expression and stimulates fibroblast proliferation
Receptors	Both bind to the same high-affinity receptor. The degree of lysis is directly related to the amount of TNF bound to the cell. Receptor binding alone may not cause cell lysis; internalisation may be required. Not all cells binding TNF are lysed by it
Cross-reactivity	TNFα shows 79% homology in humans and mice and TNFβ 74%. There is significant cross-species activity

Antibodies may cause tumour cell lysis either by fixing complement to the tumour cell membrane (resulting in the formation of the membrane attack complex and the ultimate loss of the osmotic and biochemical integrity of the cell) or by antibody-dependent cellular cytotoxicity (ADCC) mediated by natural killer (NK) cells, killer cells, macrophages or granulocytes. In vitro, the latter has been shown to be a more efficient method of cell lysis than complement-mediated cytotoxicity, since it requires fewer antibody molecules per cell to cause cytolysis. Despite this theoretically positive outcome, the production of anti-tumour antibodies may not be beneficial in all instances (Table 13.7).

Natural Killer (NK) Cells

Our understanding of the anti-tumour activity of NK cells has been largely derived from observations made of their activity in vitro. These cells do not possess the classic form of antigen-specific receptor and are thus considered to

Table 13.7   Non-beneficial effects of anti-tumour antibody production

Nature of antibody	Effect
Blocking antibodies	These may mask antigenic determinants, preventing the recognition of the tumour cells by Tc cells
Soluble immune complexes	These may form between anti-tumour antibodies and shed tumour antigen — these suppress Tc and NK cell activity in vitro

be part of the innate immune system. Thus, NK cells may provide an initial defence against tumours at both primary and metastatic sites. In addition, the activity of NK cells is enhanced by cytokines secreted by antigen-stimulated T cells, thus providing an additional means of attack once the specific immune response has been stimulated.

In vitro, NK cells kill a range of tumour targets. However, the recognition mechanism used by these cells has not yet been fully characterised; binding appears to be mediated through certain **adhesion molecules** rather than through a classical antigen-specific receptor.

As we discussed in Chapter 5, NK cell-mediated lysis results from the release of a cytotoxic factor(s) which induces the formation of holes in the target cell membrane. This activity is considerably enhanced in the presence of interleukin-2 (IL-2) and interferon-gamma (IFNγ), cytokines which are produced by antigen-stimulated Th1 cells.

There are other effector cells capable of killing tumour targets (at least in vitro) through non-antigen-specific recognition. Natural cytotoxic (NC) cells are resistant to glucocorticoids and are stimulated by IL-3. These cells kill a slightly different range of tumour targets when compared with NK cells. Lymphokine-activated killer (LAK) cells kill a much wider spectrum of targets in vitro than NK cells. These are induced by extremely high doses of IL-2 from a heterogeneous group of cells (which includes some NK and other cell types). However, their physiological role in vivo, particularly in anti-tumour responses, is unclear.

Macrophages

Macrophages have two main roles to play in tumour immunity: antigen presentation to initiate a specific immune response, and direct cytolysis of the tumour cells. In order to exhibit cytotoxic activity, tissue macrophages must be activated first by cytokines such as IFNγ, TNF, IL-4 and granulocyte-macrophage colony-stimulating factor. Since these factors are produced by antigen-stimulated T cells, the ability of macrophages to affect tumour cell growth is largely dependent upon T cell immunity.

The precise mechanisms by which macrophages recognise and destroy tumour cells are not fully understood. Attachment is energy-dependent and is brought about by trypsin-sensitive membrane receptors. Lysis may result from the intercellular transfer of lysosomal products, the production of superoxide, the release of neutral proteases or secretion of TNF, the effective mechanism being influenced by the cytokines which activated the macrophage.

Tumour Cell Evasion of the Immune Response

Tumours have been shown to possess the capability to avoid detection or destruction by the immune system (Table 13.8).

The poor, or ineffective, immune response which occurs with particular tumours may be due to selective pressures within the tumour causing a reduction in (or loss of) expression of a tumour antigen which might be capable of stimulating a good immune response (**immunoselection**). Such cells would not stimulate an antigen-specific response and thus would be unlikely to be recognised and destroyed. In other words, these tumour cells possess a selective advantage which allows them to form the dominant population; the resulting tumour is relatively resistant to immune attack.

Antigenic modulation (which is typically caused by antibodies) occurs when the immune response to a tumour antigen causes the loss of expression of that antigen. This process is similar to immunoselection, except that when the immune response is 'switched off', the antigen will be re-expressed.

Antibodies have been implicated in other ways. Patients with progressive tumours have been shown to have circulating blocking factors in their serum that inhibit tumour-specific cell-mediated cytotoxicity and ADCC. Such blocking or masking factors have been shown to be antibodies. However, it is likely that other molecules may mediate a similar effect. Certainly, circulating antigen or antigen-antibody complexes, when in excess, may block antigen-specific receptors and may alter the immune response by redirecting effector cells to non-tumour sites.

Some tumour cells themselves can release soluble suppressor factors which directly or indirectly inhibit the normal immune response. Such factors may activate certain cells of the immune system, causing them to produce cytokines

Table 13.8 Mechanisms of tumour cell evasion of the immune response

Mechanism
Immunoselection
Antigenic modulation
Production of suppressor factors

or other factors which may prevent the development of effective anti-tumour responses. Indeed, macrophages from individuals with progressive tumours are immunosuppressive, an effect which appears to be mediated through the production of prostaglandins.

CANCER BIOTHERAPY

In the last few decades, cancer therapy has advanced considerably. Many cancers are now completely curable either by chemotherapy or by a combination of surgery and chemotherapy. Unfortunately, many others remain difficult to just control, let alone cure. Modern treatments for cancers include the use of tumour vaccines, biological response modifiers, chemotherapy and radiotherapy, adoptive cellular immunotherapy and affinity column apheresis.

Tumour Vaccines

The production of tumour vaccines has relied to a great extent on the technology used to develop vaccines against infectious agents. The immunogen is usually composed of cells derived from the patient's own tumour. However, in some cases, cells from a similar but allogenic tumour are used to prepare the vaccine. Prior to inoculation, the cells are treated to prevent division and may be modified by the use of enzymes, chemicals or radiation to increase the expression of tumour-specific antigens. Alternatively, tumour-specific antigens are isolated from the cells and inoculated, often with an **adjuvant** such as BCG, to enhance the response to the antigens.

Although the technique is well established, many tumour-specific vaccines have not affected the tumour load. This may be due to a number of factors, including immune defects in tumour-bearing patients; tumour vaccines only stimulate weak responses, resulting in immunoselection.

Anti-idiotypic Antibodies

Monoclonal antibodies specific for tumour antigens have been used to stimulate the production of anti-idiotypic antibodies. Some of the latter may be able to stimulate a strong anti-tumour immune response when inoculated into the tumour-bearing patient. Thus, the anti-idiotypes must be screened for those which possess this capability before being used in a clinical setting. Although this technique is potentially very attractive, it is limited by the need to develop the anti-idiotypes in animals. The immune system of the patient being inoculated will recognise the anti-idiotypes as foreign protein and will respond rapidly, leading to the clearance of the antibody.

Table 13.9   Therapeutic effects of IFNα in cancer patients

Effect
Induces prolonged remission in chronic, progressive, hairy cell leukaemia
Induces remission in particular lymphomas and chronic myelogenous leukaemia
Slows the progression of certain solid tumours, e.g. melanoma

Adoptive Cellular Immunotherapy

Recently, a technique has been developed which entails cancer patients being inoculated with their own tumour cells which have been transfected in vitro with genes which code for immunoregulatory molecules such as IL-2 and TNFα. The theory proposes that these transfected cells will stimulate the immune response and lead to the activation of tumour-specific T cell-mediated immunity. The transfection procedure has proved to be difficult in some instances, but preliminary observations suggest that this technique may prove beneficial for certain cancers.

Biological Response Modifiers (BRM)

One of the first biological response modifiers used in the treatment of cancer was IFNα (Table 13.9). It probably exerts its effects directly on the tumour cells (possibly by inducing their re-differentiation) rather than by boosting the immune response.

   Indeed, an analogue of vitamin A — transretinoic acid — has been shown to have a similar effect to IFNα in **acute promyelocytic leukaemia**. It appears to induce the re-differentiation of the cancer cells by inhibiting the release of growth factors from activated immune cells.

LEARNING OUTCOMES

Having read this chapter you should have an idea of some of the causes of tumours and the way in which the immune system responds to them or may be encouraged to combat them. It is important to realise that tumours may arise in any tissue, may be caused by a variety of stimuli and may show totally different characteristics in different individuals. There are a huge number of different documented tumours and it is impossible to give the subject appropriate coverage in an introductory text. What I hope it has done is to give you enough information to make you read more widely in order to get a deeper understanding of this complex subject.

Chapter 14

The Immunology of Reproduction

LEARNING OBJECTIVES

The aim of this chapter is to familiarise you with the role of the immune system in reproduction. Reproduction requires the immune system of the female host to accept what is, in essence, a **foreign graft**. Advances in our understanding of the processes involved have led to the development of new approaches to the treatment of spontaneous abortion and primary infertility.

The following should give you an insight into the mechanisms involved in reproductive immunology. The references quoted are review articles and papers covering specific areas of the field and are intended as a source of further information for those who are interested.

THE DEVELOPMENT OF MATERNAL AND FETAL TISSUES

Fertilisation occurs high up in the Fallopian tube and the fertilised egg (known as the **blastocyst**) passes into the uterus, where it implants. During this stage, most of the cells formed make up the membranes which surround the embryo and provide protection and nutrition.

The wall of the blastocyst consists of an inner cellular layer, the **cytotrophoblast** (or cellular trophoblast), and an outer layer, the **syncytial trophoblast**. The latter destroys the epithelium and underlying stroma of the uterus, allowing the blastocyst to implant. At implantation, the syncytial trophoblast stimulates an inflammatory reaction which results in the formation of the **decidua**—a highly specialised tissue with the capacity to produce endocrine hormones. It derives from the **uterine endometrium**, and, under the influence of female hormones, proliferates. After implantation, it becomes thick, spongy and highly vascularised.

In early gestation, the trophoblast invades the maternal decidua and proliferates within it. This contact with the fetus is maintained throughout gestation, the decidua giving the fetus the ability to absorb nutriment from the

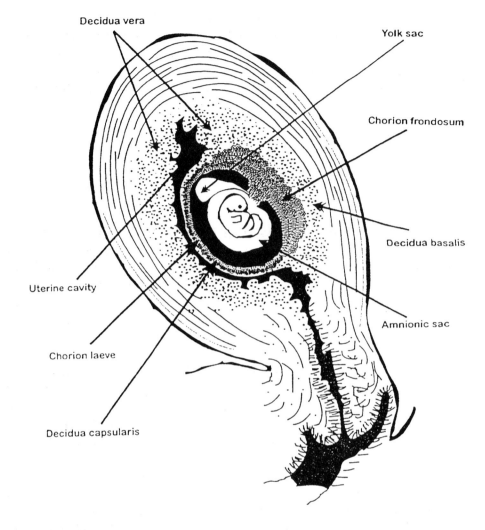

Figure 14.1   Structure of the human decidua

mother. The decidua consists of three layers: the **decidua basalis** (in which the fetus implants); the **decidua capsularis** (which lies over the fetus) and the **decidua vera** (Figure 14.1). The decidua basalis forms the maternal part of the **haemochorial placenta**. Thus, the decidua provides the contact between the mother and the fetus.

FEMALE REPRODUCTIVE IMMUNOLOGY

Half the chromosome complement of the fetus is derived from the father, and molecules coded for by paternal genes could theoretically be recognised as foreign by the maternal immune system. Thus, the fetus could be seen as a foreign tissue graft and rejected. Elsewhere in the body, transplants which are not MHC-matched are rejected as a result of the activity of cytotoxic T cells. However, despite having direct contact with the mother's blood supply, the syncytial trophoblast is not recognised by maternal cytotoxic T cells. Two principal mechanisms have been proposed which may prevent rejection of the fetus:

1. *The mother's immune response is altered in some way so that it does not respond to the stimulus.*

2. *Fetal tissues only express low levels of MHC antigens so that either the foreign (fetal) antigens are unable to stimulate the mother's immune response or they are able to induce low-dose tolerance.*

Several studies have demonstrated that syncytial trophoblast cells do not express MHC Class I antigens, which may account for the lack of fetal antigen recognition by the mother's immune system. However, maternal lymphocytes are capable of killing cultured human trophoblast cells from their own placenta, suggesting that trophoblast cells do display some transplantation antigens. In addition, fetal cells express other unique antigens (as evidenced by the production of maternal antibodies to fetal antigens) and so other factors must help to prevent fetal rejection.

The first exposure of the female to paternal antigens occurs after sexual intercourse. Although sperm bear foreign antigens, they are not recognised by the female's immune system and so are not destroyed. This may be due to **non-specific suppressor factors** in the semen. Indeed, high molecular weight substances found in seminal plasma have been shown to inhibit antigen-, mitogen- and alloantigen-stimulated lymphoproliferation.

Rejection of the fetus (which results from recognition of paternal antigens expressed on the placenta and trophoblast) may be prevented by gestational steroid and protein hormones. Although the concentration of these substances is never great enough in the maternal serum to suppress immunity in vivo, together they may exert a potent immunosuppressive effect at the fetal–maternal interface, where they are maintained at high levels during most stages of pregnancy. The trophoblast produces most of the major pregnancy-associated hormones shown to be capable of altering the maternal immune response.

MATERNAL–FETAL EXCHANGE

Although the fetus and mother are separated, cells and soluble substances can pass through the placenta during gestation, particularly at the time of placental separation. Syncytial trophoblast cells are continuously released from the placenta and, from the 18th week of gestation, can be found circulating in the mother's blood. Thus, the placenta only forms a partial barrier to the passage of cells and molecules between the mother and the fetus. It is thought that the recognition of fetal antigens by the mother's immune system may result from this passage of cells, and this is thought to protect the mother from the extensive and otherwise unchecked growth and invasion of the trophoblast, as occurs in **choriocarcinoma**.

The only class of antibody readily transferred from the mother to the fetus is IgG. This transference is probably mediated by Fc receptors on the surface of placental cells. Unless infection occurs in utero, the newborn cannot mount a quick, effective response to pathogenic organisms, and the transplacentally acquired maternal antibody is the only protection a baby has against infection for the first 6–8 months of its life.

In certain circumstances, maternal antibody is not beneficial to the fetus, e.g. **haemolytic disease of the newborn**. This disease is due to incompatible blood groups in the mother and fetus and occurs primarily in blood group O mothers carrying a fetus with group A or B blood. It is thought to result from the transfer of IgG antibodies (from mother to fetus) which react with the fetal erythrocyte antigens. Although women of group A or group B have antibody to type B and type A erythrocytes, respectively, these natural antibodies are usually of the IgM class and therefore do not readily cross the placenta and cannot harm the fetus.

A more important complication which affects fetal development involves the **rhesus (Rh) antigens**, which are expressed only on blood cells; antigenic determinants of the A and B blood groups are widely distributed in nature and in the human body. During pregnancy, if a Rh-negative mother is carrying a Rh-positive fetus, fetal erythrocytes can cross the placenta and stimulate the production of antibodies to the Rh antigen in the maternal circulation. If this is untreated, in subsequent pregnancies this antibody may cross the placenta and lyse the erythrocytes of any Rh-positive fetus. Anti-rhesus antibodies may also be formed in the mother if there is transplacental haemorrhage at birth or after an abortion. Lysis of fetal red blood cells can be prevented by giving the mother **anti-Rho(D) antiserum** immediately after delivery of her first Rh-positive child or following an abortion. Any fetal erythrocytes present in the mother's circulation are destroyed by the passively administered antibody and are rapidly cleared. In this way, they are not present long enough to sensitise the mother effectively.

EFFECT OF PREGNANCY ON THE MATERNAL IMMUNE RESPONSE

Pregnancy is associated with a depression in cellular immunity which may result from a change in the number and function of T cells. Peripheral blood total lymphocyte counts fall during gestation and this is associated with a decrease in T cell numbers. Towards the end of pregnancy, CD4+ cells decrease and

CD8+ cells increase. In addition, circulating NK cell numbers decline during pregnancy but their level of activity is probably unchanged. In vitro tests of T cell function, using mitogens and mixed lymphocyte reactions, show a decrease in lymphoproliferation during pregnancy. Serum immunoglobulin concentrations increase, but alterations of specific immunoglobulin subclasses have not been well characterised.

Immunity to Infection in Pregnancy

Perhaps not surprisingly, pregnant women are at increased risk of acquiring those infectious diseases primarily controlled by **cell-mediated immunity**. The pregnancy-related alteration in the immune response in infection includes changes in T cell subpopulations, neutrophil function, lymphocyte function, serum immunoglobulin concentrations, immunosuppressive serum factors and maternal immune-recognition mechanisms. A number of infectious agents are thought to behave differently in pregnant women as a result of the altered immune response. These include viruses (e.g. cytomegalovirus (CMV), Epstein–Barr virus (EBV), influenza A virus), bacteria (e.g. *Neisseria gonorrhoeae, Streptococcus pneumoniae*) and fungi. Changes in the humoral immune response may play a role in this increased susceptibility. Serum IgG concentration decreases with advancing gestation. A decrease in the levels of IgM and IgM-bearing lymphocytes has also been reported in the first trimester, but these levels do not continue to decrease with advancing gestation. Antibody production in response to infection during pregnancy is probably unaltered. A number of factors have been implicated in the decrease in cell-mediated immunity seen in pregnancy. These include the **steroid hormones** produced in pregnancy, such as progesterone, oestrogens, cortisol, α-fetoprotein and uromodulin. Despite this range of changes in immune reactivity, the human fetus usually remains relatively unaffected by maternal infectious diseases. However, there are some infectious agents which may have serious effects if the foetus is exposed during the early stages of its development. These include rubella, CMV, syphilis and toxoplasmosis.

IMMUNOCOMPETENT CELLS IN THE DECIDUA

Many of the cells comprising the decidua have immunological activity and are thought to release **immunomodulatory factors** which help to ensure the survival of the fetus.

Large Granular Lymphocytes

Studies on the cellular constituents of human first trimester decidua have shown that the largest population of cells are non-T, non-B, large granular lymphocytes. The majority express CD56 (the peripheral blood natural killer (NK) cell marker), whilst approximately 9% lack CD56 and NK cell activity but express CD16, the FcγRIII receptor. In mice, these CD16+, decidual large granular lymphocytes produce a suppressor factor (100 kDa) which inhibits cytotoxic T lymphocyte responses in both primary and secondary mixed lymphocyte cultures through the inhibition of lymphocyte responses to interleukin-2.

Macrophages

Macrophages constitute approximately 14% of the immunocompetent cells in decidua. In addition to CD14, the majority of these cells express the MHC Class II antigens HLA-DR, HLA-DP or HLA-DQ. Enzymatically released decidual macrophages have been shown to suppress mixed lymphocyte responses and alloreactive cytotoxic T cell activity in vitro. The molecule responsible for this suppression was shown to be **prostaglandin E_2 (PGE$_2$)**, since the effect could be wiped out by adding anti-PGE$_2$ antibody or indomethacin to the cultures.

Decidual Antigen-presenting Cells

Antigen-presenting cells from the decidua have been shown to be capable of stimulating the generation of CD8+ suppressor T cells specific for antigens expressed on villous chorion and fetal cells to which the antigen-presenting cells were exposed in vitro. These T cells were capable of inhibiting allogeneic mixed lymphocyte reactions and the development of antigen-specific cytotoxic T cells. This suggests that, unlike a peripheral immune response, that in the decidua is geared towards suppression (or tolerance) rather than to the elimination of an invader.

T Lymphocytes

Immunocytochemical studies have demonstrated that approximately 10–20% of decidual mononuclear cells are T lymphocytes. Since the expression of the TCR–CD3 complex on these cells has been found to be extremely low, it has been suggested that this may be responsible for the lack of demonstrable fetal antigen recognition.

In women undergoing natural spontaneous abortion, the percentage of CD3+ HLA-DR+ T cells in the decidua has been shown to be increased. Since only activated T cells express HLA-DR, it is possible that these cells may play an active role in fetal rejection.

SUPPRESSIVE FACTORS IN DECIDUA

There are a wide variety of documented changes in the immune system of the pregnant, compared to the non-pregnant, female. Whilst a number of naturally occurring substances have been shown to exhibit immunosuppressive capabilities e.g. α-**fetoprotein**, **antibody**, **steroid** and **protein hormones**, there is no direct evidence to suggest that these factors alone are responsible for the modulation observed.

Prostaglandins

Decidual macrophages have been shown to secrete prostaglandin E_2, a molecule with potent immunosuppressive activity. However, the role of this factor in vivo is unclear, since only those cells isolated by enzymatic methods appeared to secrete PGE_2.

Transforming Growth Factor-beta

One factor isolated from the decidua which is capable of causing suppression has a molecular mass of 60–100 kDa. Under acid isolation conditions the suppressive activity was associated with a molecule of 13 kDa. The decidua factor inhibited IL-2-dependent cytotoxic T lymphocyte responses but did not block the binding of radiolabelled IL-2 to the IL-2 receptor. A specific antibody to transforming growth factor-beta (TGFβ) eliminated this activity. TGFβ is a dimeric protein of 25 kDa. This active protein is derived from a latent form which consists of two large polypeptide chains linked via a disulphide bond to the latent TGFβ-binding protein (LTBP). This complex has a molecular mass of approximately 210 kDa. However, since the size of the LTBP varies depending upon the cell from which it is produced, the latent complex can show a wide variation in molecular mass. The transforming growth factor family consists of a number of structurally related molecules with important regulatory activity in cell growth and tissue development.

TGFβ is produced by most of the cells which have been examined. The active species, which is cleaved from the latent complex, interacts with three main cell surface receptors; one is β-glycan and the other two are serine and threonine kinases. Originally isolated as a growth promoter, TGFβ may act as a growth inhibitor also. It tends to inhibit the growth of lymphoid, epithelial and endothelial cells and to promote the formation of collagen, fibronectin and certain proteoglycans. In the pregnant female it has been suggested that TGFβ limits the invasion of the fetal tissues into the maternal decidua. However, it may also play a role in 'damping down' any local immunological response to fetal antigens.

Table 14.1   Characteristics of the transforming growth factors

Characteristic	Type	Information
Molecular mass	α	6 kDa (human); 6 kDa (rat)
	β	44.3 kDa (human TGFβ1); 47.8 kDa (human TGFβ2); 47.3 kDa (human TGFβ3)
Major cellular	α	Monocytes, keratinocytes and many tissues and tumours
sources	β	Platelets contain TGFβ1 and TGFβ2. Most nucleated cell types and many tumours express TGFβ1, TGFβ2, TGFβ3 or combinations thereof
Effects	α	Can act as a self-inductive growth factor. Shares biological and structural properties with epidermal growth factor.
	β	Integral membrane protein. Involved in tissue remodelling, wound repair, development and haematopoiesis. Inhibits cell growth. Switch factor for IgA
Cross-reactivity	α	Structurally related to endothelial growth factor (EGF) and vaccinia growth factor, both of which bind to the EGF receptor. Active across species
	β	TGFβ species show greater than 98% homology in humans and mice

Tumour Necrosis Factor

Decidual stromal cells and macrophages are capable of producing the lymphokine tumour necrosis factor (TNFα). TNF has a similar range of activities to interleukin-1 (IL-1) and can stimulate the proliferation of T and B cells and (along with interferon-gamma (IFNγ)) can cause the up-regulation of HLA-DR antigen expression. TNF has been shown to be present in amniotic fluid and in the supernatant of human decidual cell culture. It has been suggested that this lymphokine may affect fetal survival during early pregnancy.

RECURRENT, SPONTANEOUS, ABORTION

In order for the mother to recognise and accept the fetus, it is thought that an **allogeneic incompatibility** is necessary at an HLA or closely linked locus. If this incompatibility is not present, the fetus may be rejected by cell-mediated or humoral reactions. Recurrent, spontaneous abortion has been shown to be more common in couples who share certain HLA specificities.

The **minor histocompatibility antigens** TA1 and TLX appear to be important in preventing recognition of fetally expressed paternal antigens. If these antigens are not matched in the male and female, the pregnant female may recognise the paternal TLX as foreign, thereby being stimulated to produce an immune response. This may result in the production of an antibody that prevents a response to the foreign TA1, thus preventing rejection. If mates are matched for TLX, the maternal immune system cannot recognise the paternal TLX antigen, and antibody which prevents a response to TA1 will not be produced. Thus, an immune response to TA1 may occur, leading to rejection of the fetus.

THE IMMUNOLOGY OF MALE REPRODUCTION

Since the male immune system is not exposed to antigens from the female during intercourse, any immunological abnormalities affecting the male reproductive system are likely to be **autoimmune**. Autoimmune recognition of sperm antigens is frequently reported in infertile couples and in individuals who have undergone vasectomy. Normally, antibodies which recognise determinants on the sperm surface are not found in the sera of healthy males or females; their presence indicates an unusual immune response which may affect the function of the spermatozoa. In contrast to this, antibodies directed towards **spermatozoan cytoplasmic antigens** have been demonstrated in 90% of sera from children of both sexes before puberty. The incidence declines to about 60% and thereafter persists throughout life.

> The genital tracts of female rabbits have been shown to contain sperm, the head regions of which are coated with antibody. The antibody was bound by a receptor found only on non-motile sperm and those that appeared to be dying. It has been suggested that this antibody may be important in the removal of spermatozoa from the female reproductive tract.

The Blood–Testis Barrier

During development, the male immune system may not be tolerised to sperm-specific antigens, owing to the fact that they are sequestered behind a **blood–testis barrier**. However, this same barrier may be effective enough to prevent subsequent development of autoimmune diseases affecting the sperm or testicular cells by maintaining a partition between the spermatozoa and the host immune system. Unfortunately, evidence exists to suggest that this barrier is not totally exclusive, since some sperm-specific antigens have been detected in the seminiferous tubules. Reaction to these antigens may be prevented in a number of ways, e.g. suppressor cells, non-specific suppressive mechanisms, lack of antigen presentation and lack of lymphocyte trafficking through the testes.

Sperm-specific Antigens

HLA antigens have not been demonstrated on the surface of spermatozoa. Anti-sperm antibodies appear to recognise tissue-specific antigens, since they react with sperm from individuals with different HLA antigens.

> Since tolerisation to spermatozoa does not normally occur, vasectomy may lead to exposure of the immune system to sperm-associated antigens and the development of autoimmune disease. An association has been demonstrated between the expression of HLA-A28 and the development of anti-sperm antibodies in vasectomised men. These antibodies have been shown to form circulating immune complexes which, in monkeys, have been implicated in the rapid onset of atherosclerosis.

Immunologically Active Cells in Semen

Immunologically active cells have been demonstrated in the semen of healthy men. CD8+ suppressor T lymphocytes which have been demonstrated in the epithelium of the epididymis are thought to prevent autoimmune reactions by controlling local B cell differentiation and production of anti-sperm antibody. Alternatively, these suppressor cells may suppress local antigen processing and presentation by macrophages.

LEARNING OUTCOMES

The special relationship between the mother and fetus presents an interesting scenario in which to test our understanding of immune responses. Some of the antigens expressed by the fetus are foreign but you should now understand why immune responses which would cause the rejection of the fetus do not normally take place. You should have a working knowledge of the most common factors which are thought to prevent or damp down the immune response in the pregnant female and the autoimmune responses which may result in male sterility. You should explore this subject further using the reading material suggested in the Further Reading.

Chapter 15

Transplantation

LEARNING OBJECTIVES

The first successful human organ transplantation was a cadaveric renal graft (kidney transplant) carried out in 1954. Although early operations were often unsuccessful due to fatal post-operative infections and rejection of the transplanted organ, by the 1960s the development of immunosuppressive drugs such as **prednisolone** and **azathioprine** caused a significant reduction in rejection and mortality rates. This pioneering work led to the refinement of techniques which allowed the successful transplantation of hearts, livers, lungs and bone marrow. Other transplantation techniques such as for heart–lung and bowel are becoming more successful as we understand the nature of the rejection reaction and how to prevent or control it. This chapter is designed to give you an understanding of the mechanisms involved in organ transplantation and rejection and how they can be regulated to allow successful transplantation. We will consider each of the major transplant organs in turn, highlighting the aspects of the process which are peculiar to that organ.

KIDNEY TRANSPLANTATION

Patients with 'end-state' renal disease may be considered for organ transplant only when all other options have been exhausted. The patient must not be suffering from certain diseases which affect the heart or lungs, cancer, peptic ulcers, or diseases or infections which complicate the use of anaesthetics or immunosuppressive therapy. If these criteria are fulfilled, the patient is 'tissue typed' so that a suitable (matching) organ may be found. This process of tissue typing involves **ABO blood typing, human leukocyte antigen (HLA) typing** and determining if the patient is **pre-sensitised** by testing for pre-existing antibodies to HLA. When a suitable organ is obtained, the degree of **haplotype matching** (i.e. identity between the recipient and donor for major human leukocyte antigens) must be determined.

In addition to being present on red blood cells, blood group antigens (the ABO antigens) are also expressed on the endothelium lining the blood vessels (vascular endothelium) of a graft. Thus, in order to prevent its rejection by the recipient's immune system, the blood type of the grafted kidney must be compatible with that of the recipient. If the organ and recipient are not matched, rapid rejection occurs due to the presence of natural antibodies directed against blood group antigens (isohaemagglutinins). These damage the vascular endothelium, causing localised coagulation, reduced blood circulation through the transplanted organ and anoxia (oxygen lack). The outcome is widespread cytotoxicity, massive tissue damage and rapid organ rejection.

Clearly, it is important that the HLA antigens of the donor and recipient are matched as closely as possible, since it is these antigens that mediate immune recognition of foreign antigens and, if foreign to the host, will act as the focus of an immune response. In grafted tissue, this would present as a **rejection reaction**. However, despite the complexity of the process, the survival of patients after renal transplantation is similar to that of patients undergoing dialysis.

Related-donor Transplantation

The relatives of patients awaiting kidney transplantation may be assessed for their suitability as donors. Such close genetic relatedness between the recipient and donor gives the transplant a greater chance of success. Indeed, studies have shown that when the recipient and donor are siblings with two matching haplotypes, the graft survival rate after 1 year is 90%. One-haplotype-matched pairs (the organ being from either a sibling or a parent) have a 75–85% graft survival rate after 1 year. This rate declines to only 50–60% in zero-haplotype-matched family members unless the recipient receives some form of immunosuppressive or modulatory treatment such as **transfusion therapy**. Studies have shown that transfusion therapy is beneficial in related-donor transplantation where the donor and recipient share none, or only one, haplotype. Obviously, this technique allows the identification of those recipients in whom transplantation is contraindicated due to their ability to immunologically recognise the donor tissue. Not so obvious is the way in which transfusion therapy improves the survival rate of grafts in those individuals who do not recognise the foreign antigens. It has been suggested that a number of mechanisms (including clonal deletion, selection of immunological non-responders, induction of suppressor T cells or the production of blocking or anti-idiotypic antibodies) may act individually or in concert.

Transfusion therapy usually consists of three transfusions of small amounts (100–200 ml) of donor blood given over a period of several weeks. The production of cytotoxic anti-donor antibodies (which occurs in approximately 10–30% of recipients) is carefully monitored. In most donor–recipient pairs matched for only one haplotype, anti-donor antibody production can be reduced by the use of azathioprine during the transfusions. In those individuals who do not become sensitised to the donor during this therapy, 2-year survival rates in one-haplotype-matched related-donor transplantations are 95%. Indeed, pre-transplant transfusion treatment has resulted in greatly improved survival rates in non-haplotype-matched allografts (> 90% at 2 years).

Pre-sensitisation

Organ donation by relatives, whilst having a greater chance for success, also allows for the possibility of pre-sensitisation. Previous exposure to transplantation antigens (e.g. in women who have had multiple pregnancies) can lead to the development of **HLA-specific antibodies** which may cause rejection of subsequent grafts bearing those antigens. Similarly, patients receiving more than one transplant are more likely to undergo a rejection reaction than patients receiving a single graft. In addition, a patient undergoing rapid rejection of a primary graft (in less than 3 months) is much more likely to reject a subsequent graft.

The risk of rejection of the graft is assessed using a technique known as the mixed lymphocyte culture (MLC). White cells from the donor are treated to prevent them from proliferating. These are then mixed with white cells from the recipient. If the MHC antigens on the donor cells are different to those on the recipient cells, they will be recognised as foreign and the recipient cell will be stimulated by them and proliferate. The stronger the proliferative reaction, the more likely that the graft will be rejected. However, the degree of proliferation does not necessarily correlate with the degree of matching between the donor and recipient, since some antigens are much stronger stimulators than others. Thus, different donor–recipient pairs matched for a single haplotype may show distinct graft survival rates due to the immunogenicity of the non-matched antigens.

The presence of pre-formed antibodies to HLAs is detected by cross-matching. A serum sample taken from the potential recipient is mixed with lymphocytes from a range of different people. The number of cell cultures that show cytotoxicity is expressed as a percentage of that panel. If those cells bearing antigens present in the proposed graft tissue are destroyed, the transplantation is unlikely to be successful.

If an appropriate donor is found, improved methods of **pre-operative conditioning** and better **immunosuppressive therapy** regimes have greatly increased the success rates of related-donor transplantation (Table 15.1). Indeed, it is now possible to consider living donors who share two, one or even no haplotypes with the recipient. Some studies have suggested that living, unrelated donors may also be considered, provided that appropriate pre-operative conditioning procedures are followed.

In individuals who have donated a kidney for transplantation there appears to be no long-term change in survival or lifestyle. The procedure requires that not only is the kidney removed, but also all the renal arteries and veins and the ureter with all the associated periureteral soft tissue. The latter ensures that an intact ureteral blood supply is available, thus preventing necrosis of the ureter.

Cadaveric Kidney Transplantation

In some cases, an appropriate relative for organ donation cannot be found and the recipient must receive an organ from a recently deceased individual. After screening, but before transplantation, patients receiving a kidney transplant from a non-related individual are pre-conditioned; this can include a range of techniques. For patients awaiting cadaveric transplantation, it has been found

Table 15.1 Examples of immunosuppressive agents used post-operatively

Agent	Effects
Cyclosporine (5–15 mg/kg/day)	Has enhanced allograft survival in recipients of both cadaveric and related-donor transplants
Cyclosporine	Has received widespread use but is nephrotoxic, and doses and in vivo levels must be carefully monitored
Azathioprine	An anti-metabolite that interferes with DNA formation in proliferating cells. Often used in combination with prednisolone and cyclosporine. Potentially hepatotoxic
Cyclophosphamide	Used as a non-hepatotoxic alternative to azathioprine
Anti-lymphocyte (ALG) or anti-thymocyte globulin (ATG). Therapeutic dose: 10–20 mg/kg	Polyclonal antisera prepared in animals immunised with human lymphocytes or thymocytes (respectively). The cytolytic activity of the antibodies results in profound immunosuppression
Lymphoplasmapheresis	Used concurrently, occasionally, with immunosuppressive drugs to remove recipient lymphocytes and immunoglobulin

that pre-operative, random blood transfusion is correlated with improved allograft survival. Although as little as 1 unit of random blood has been shown to be effective, the larger the number of transfusions, the better the graft survival. This transfusion treatment means that individuals who will produce cytotoxic, blocking or anti-idiotypic antibodies, and specific or non-specific suppressor T cells, can be identified. Transplantation is not suitable for such individuals.

Repeated exposure to the foreign HLAs encourages the formation of specific antibodies (if the recipient is prone to it) which are detected by repeated screening. This determines the extent of pre-sensitisation of the recipient (i.e. the potential frequency of positive cross-matches between donor and recipient, assuming that the transplant organ is taken from the same genetic pool of donors as the lymphocyte panel). The cell panel usually consists of between 40 and 50 samples, thus allowing for the majority of HLAs to be represented twice.

When a potential donor is identified (and after permission is obtained from the next of kin), organs which are likely to be useful for transplantation are removed and a section of the spleen, some lymph nodes and some peripheral blood are collected. The latter are used for blood group and HLA typing of the donor.

ABO-compatible recipients who are cross-match negative are subjected to further cross-match testing using additional past sera to eliminate the possibility of undetected pre-sensitisation. The best-matched recipients are selected and further criteria are taken into consideration, such as the urgency of their medical condition, the length of time on the waiting list and whether they have received a previous transplant.

As with living donor organs, the kidneys are removed with the renal arteries and veins, as well as the ureters and periureteral soft tissue intact. However, cadaveric organs usually also have the donor aorta and vena cava attached. Once removed, the kidney must be cleaned (to remove all donor blood) and cooled (to help its preservation). This is achieved by flushing it through with a **mixed-electrolyte solution**. The kidneys are stored until transplantation (preferably for no more than 48 hours) by one of two methods: (a) cold storage (which involves packing the organ in ice to maintain subphysiological temperatures); (b) pulsed, cold perfusion with mixed-electrolyte solution by cannulation of the aorta or renal arteries.

Rejection

Rejection of a transplanted organ may present as **acute**, **hyperacute** or **chronic**. Each is associated with particular signs and symptoms which are related to the underlying immunological mechanisms causing the rejection. Classical acute rejection of kidney transplants presents as swelling and tenderness over the allograft and decreased renal function (decreased urine volume and increased blood urea, nitrogen and creatinine levels). In addition, patients may present with elevated temperature, malaise, decreased appetite and generalised myalgia.

Mechanisms Involved in Acute Rejection

In the early stages post-transplantation, most of the cells invading the graft tissue are lymphocytes. However, 4–7 days after transplantation the tissue contains a heterogeneous collection of cells. Evidence suggests that early rejection of solid grafts is caused by cytotoxic T cells, although initiation of the reaction is thought to be mediated by '**passenger cells**' in the graft. These are dendritic cells and MHC Class II-expressing monocytes capable of producing IL-1 and IL-2 which help to trigger lymphocyte activation. Alloantigens on the graft stimulate the activation of T cells, leading to the development of specific, cellular immune responses. Once activated, these cells release IL-2, which stimulates the proliferation and maturation of alloantigen-specific cells, leading to the development of both CD4 + and CD8 + effector T cells. The latter circulate from the lymphoid tissue through the vascular system to the graft, where they cause antigen-specific damage, either directly or by stimulating the release of cytotoxic antibodies. In addition, stimulated Th1 cells produce interferon-γ (IFNγ), which has been shown to have a variety of effects which enhance graft rejection (Table 15.2).

By contrast, stimulation of Th2 cells leads to the production of IL-4 and IL-5, which promote the proliferation and differentiation of B cells capable of recognising graft-specific antigens. The resultant antibody causes cytolytic damage to the graft, either through the activation of complement or by mediating antibody-dependent cell-mediated cytotoxicity. When the host has been primed to donor antigens before transplantation, a more rapid effect may occur, often marked by antibody-mediated vasculitis.

During acute rejection, an increased proportion of CD4 + cells has been observed in the peripheral circulation, although many studies have suggested

Table 15.2   Effect of IFNγ in kidney transplantation

Effects of IFNγ	Consequences of effects
IFNγ enhances the expression of MHC Class I and Class II antigens on the cells of the graft	Increased MHC antigen expression may increase the effectiveness of graft-specific cytotoxic T cells
IFNγ activates macrophages both within and around the graft	Macrophage activation results in a delayed-type hypersensitivity response which gives rise to the characteristic symptoms of inflammation associated with graft rejection. In addition, the macrophages themselves may express enhanced cytotoxic activity towards the graft

that rejection is associated with an increase in CD8+ cells in the kidney. In general, it is considered to be indicative that rejection may be reversible with therapy if the peripheral blood CD4/CD8 ratio is >1.0.

Mechanisms Involved in Hyperacute Rejection

Hyperacute rejection of a graft is caused by a type II hypersensitivity response initiated by the presence of anti-ABO isohaemagglutinins or antibodies to MHC Class I antigens. When present in high enough concentration, these antibodies bind to the vascular endothelium, thus initiating the fixation and activation of the complement cascade. The sequelae include activation of the clotting pathway and, if the reaction is great enough, formation of microthrombi which block the capillaries of the graft, preventing blood flow (ischaemia) and causing necrosis of the graft. Currently, hyperacute rejection cannot be reversed once it has started.

Mechanisms Involved in Chronic Rejection

Chronic rejection, which can occur months or even years after transplantation, is characterised by proliferation of the endothelial cells lining the blood vessels of the graft, which leads to a narrowing of the lumen. The precipitating signal for this reaction is unknown but it is likely to be caused by the release of IL-1 from monocytes and platelet-derived growth factor from platelets and endothelial cells. In the initial stages, this condition is reversible with immunosuppressive therapy. However, once the changes have become fibrotic, the condition becomes progressive, leading to ischaemia and, ultimately, loss of function of the grafted tissue.

LIVER TRANSPLANTATION

Although initially unsuccessful when first attempted in 1963, liver transplantation has become more successful with the development of improved methods of immunosuppression. Originally considered to be an immunologically privileged site, transplanted livers are now known to be susceptible to immunological responses. However, rejection reactions in liver transplant patients are clearly distinct to those observed in kidney and other whole organ transplant patients.

The most common cause of liver damage requiring transplantation is chronic active non-A, non-B, viral hepatitis. However, liver transplantation has also been performed in individuals with primary biliary cirrhosis, hepatitis B, cirrhosis, and inborn errors of metabolism. Patients with progressive liver disease may present with a variety of symptoms, including malaise, weight loss, encephalopathy, raised serum albumin and bilirubin levels and renal insufficiency. Such individuals are considered suitable transplant recipients if they have a life-expectancy of less than 2 years.

Post-transplantation infection is common and patient survival is related to the type of infectious agent involved. In general, bacterial infections respond well to antibiotic therapy whilst fungal or viral infections are associated with a poor prognosis.

Procedure

Clearly, the range of organs which can be donated by living family members without endangering their life is limited. Thus, patients requiring transplantation of major organs such as the heart, lung, bowel or liver receive them from individuals who are recently deceased. Livers for transplantation are usually matched for blood group with the recipient. Generally, donor and recipient are not matched for MHC antigens and, indeed, in recent years, evidence has accumulated to suggest that there is an inverse relationship between MHC antigen matching and graft survival.

Another factor influencing liver transplantation is the size of the donor organ, although, recently, surgical reduction in the size of donor livers has changed the whole approach to this procedure in small recipients. In addition, as a consequence of this work, partial grafts from live donors may be used in liver transplantation. Since there are very few reports of hyperacute rejection due to pre-formed anti-donor antibodies, cross-matches are performed only post-operatively. The mechanisms underlying the apparent resistance of the liver to rejection are unknown; maybe the liver is not sensitive to pre-formed antibodies, or the size of the liver itself causes the dilution of the antibody to a non-pathogenic level.

After removal from the donor, the liver is flushed through with heparinised lactated Ringer's solution, immersed in preservation solution and stored in the cold. Newer preservation solutions have enabled livers to be transplanted more than 24 hours after removal from the deceased.

Primary Non-function and Rejection

Following transplantation, patients may present with a range of clinical conditions which are collectively known as primary non-function. This is really a spectrum of diseases ranging from a total lack of function of the graft (leading to death if a second transplant is not available) to a mild, initial impairment of function which corrects within the first days or weeks following transplantation. Factors which affect the development of primary non-function are listed in Table 15.3.

Histologically defined rejection reactions are seen in approximately 75% of all patients. If diagnosed early enough (through the use of frequent biopsies), they may be easily and successfully treated. However, failure of the organ a long

Table 15.3 Factors affecting the development of primary non-function in liver transplants

Factor
The nature of the donor's injury
Problems during excision of the donor organ
The type of preservation solution used
The length of organ preservation
The immunological background of the recipient
The transplantation procedure
Factors affecting the recipient's cardiovascular system

time after transplantation is usually due to chronic rejection or recurrence of the original disease. A particularly dramatic type of rejection is associated with bile duct damage, disappearance of the ducts being associated with early graft loss. Generally, liver transplants are successful, survival rates being 70–90% after 1 year and approximately 60% after 5 years.

Clinically, rejection is associated with non-specific signs and symptoms such as fever, abdominal pain, enlargement of the liver and depressed appetite. Histologically, livers undergoing rejection show a mixed cellular infiltrate with damage to the epithelium of the bile duct, and central or portal veins. Serum levels of bilirubin, alkaline phosphatase and transaminases may be abnormal but are not predictive of rejection. Treatment with a range of immunosuppressive regimes, which include either methylprednisolone, anti-lymphocyte globulin or anti-CD3 monoclonal antibody, help to prevent rejection. In addition, the use of cyclosporine post-transplantation has greatly improved survival rates.

HEART TRANSPLANTATION

Since the first successful heart transplant in 1967, the techniques used for cardiac allotransplantation have been greatly refined. This treatment is appropriate for patients with end-stage cardiac disease that has not responded to normal management techniques. However, it is contraindicated in patients with infection, severe pulmonary hypertension or cancer.

Donor organs are usually obtained only from individuals below the age of 40 without a previous history of cardiac disease. Before removal from the donor, the heart is maintained in optimal condition by hydration of the body and the carefully regulated use of vasopressor and myotropic drugs. After removal from the body, the coronary circulation is flushed with a mixed-electrolyte solution and the organ kept on ice for no more than 4 hours.

Before transplantation, the donor and recipient undergo blood group and HLA typing. Cross-matching is also performed against a random panel of lymphocytes from a number of donors. If the recipient has antibodies to more than 15% of the panel, then cross-matching with the donor must be performed before the transplantation.

Typically, acute rejection is seen as a mononuclear cell infiltrate which comprises lymphocytes, lymphoblasts and monocytes. Treatment for this condition involves the use of anti-lymphocyte globulin and/or high concentrations of corticosteroids.

BONE MARROW TRANSPLANTATION

Early attempts at bone marrow transplantation (1968) involved the infusion of marrow from human leukocyte antigen-identical siblings. Consequently, the majority of donors have been either the identical twin of the recipient (syngeneic) or an individual with an identical HLA genotype (allogeneic). However, due to the limitations of this system (only 40% of patients may have an HLA-identical donor), techniques have been developed to improve the success of marrow transplants from only partially matched family members or unrelated donors. In patients with diseases which require severe doses of chemoradiotherapy but which do not involve the bone marrow (e.g. certain types of cancer), autologous marrow transplants are indicated. This circumvents the problem of graft-versus-host disease (GVH). In addition, the marrow may be treated with monoclonal antibodies to remove potential

Graft-versus-host disease is caused by the presence of immunocompetent cells in an organ given to an immunocompromised host. It even occurs in patients who are HLA identical with their donors, the disease being attributed to minor differences in histocompatibility.

The disease presents as a skin rash associated with diarrhoea and jaundice. In severe disease, the rash resembles extensive second-degree burns and watery diarrhoea is associated with malabsorption, cramps and gastrointestinal bleeding. Hyperbilirubinaemia is often seen due to inflammation of small bile ducts as a direct consequence of the disease process. Immunocompetent CD8 + T cells are found in those tissues which have high levels of HLA-DR antigens, e.g. the skin and intestine.

Modern immunosuppressive therapy using both methotrexate and cyclosporine has reduced the risk of acute GVH disease to 25%. Established, acute GVH disease has been treated with infusions of anti-thymocyte globulin, prednisolone and monoclonal antibodies; however, success was limited. In bone marrow transplants, the donor marrow has been incubated in vitro with T cell specific monoclonal antibodies, either with complement or conjugated to toxins. These treatments decreased the incidence of GVH disease by depleting the marrow of donor T cells.

neoplastic cells, thus extending the use of this technique. There are five principal diseases that are treatable with marrow transplantation. These are severe combined immunodeficiency, aplastic anaemia, leukaemia, lymphoma and certain solid tumours.

Donor marrow is obtained in a single procedure by multiple aspirations from the top of the hip girdle (the iliac crest). Generally, 10 ml/kg of the recipient's body weight is required. The aspiration is done using heparinised needles, the marrow being placed in heparinised, buffered culture medium. The mixture is filtered through fine meshes to produce a single-cell suspension and nucleated-cell counts are obtained. Blood group-compatible recipients are given $2-6 \times 10^8$ nucleated cells/kg of body weight by intravenous infusion. Erythrocytes are given simultaneously. If the blood groups of the donor and recipient are not compatible, either the recipient undergoes plasmapheresis (to remove anti-A or anti-B antibodies) or the donor marrow is treated in vitro to remove the erythrocytes.

The immune system of most recipients must be destroyed in order to prevent rejection of the marrow and to allow the development of a new haemapoietic system.This is achieved by treating the recipient with cyclophosphamide (50–60 mg/kg, for 2 or 4 days) and by total-body irradiation (7.5–15 Gy administered over 3–5 days; a single dose of radiation would damage the lungs and eyes). This combination of therapies eliminates the immune system and has an antineoplastic effect in most cancer patients. Obviously, patients undergoing bone marrow transplantation to combat severe combined immunodeficiency disease do not require this treatment, since they lack a functioning immune system.

Success of the transplant is indicated by an increasing white cell count, raised levels of circulating monocytes (monocytosis) and the presence of mature neutrophils in the circulation between 2 and 4 weeks post-transplantation. As these parameters normalise, antibiotic therapy can be stopped and transfusions become unnecessary. Unfortunately, the technique is not always successful and GVH disease and infections are responsible for the 10–30% failure rate in the first 30 days following transplantation. Other causes of transplant failure include interstitial pneumonia, veno-occlusive liver disease and recurrence of the underlying disease.

PANCREAS TRANSPLANTATION

Pancreas transplantation is used to prevent the sequelae of diabetes, which include damage to the kidneys (nephropathy), nerves (neuropathy) and retinas (retinopathy). However, currently the procedure is only life-enhancing. Since the purpose of the procedure is to provide biologically responsive insulin-producing tissue, it may be performed with a whole organ, a segmental graft or dispersed islets of Langerhans. Recipients and donor organs are typed for both blood group and HLAs and recipients undergo cross-matching.

The survival of isolated islet cells is shorter than that of any other allograft. However, animal studies have shown that syngeneic implants in the liver or under the capsule of the kidney are able to produce insulin to reverse hyperglycaemia, so research has centred on perfecting the techniques for allograft islet transplantation. Either the adult or the fetal pancreas is used as a source of islet cells. However, the islets themselves contain dendritic cells and other antigen-presenting cells, which renders the tissue immunogenic. Attempts to reduce this effect have included treatment with antibodies to MHC Class II antigens, irradiation and culturing purified islets in an oxygen-rich atmosphere. In animal models, these techniques resulted in the correction of the diabetes. However, the clinical efficacy of these techniques remains to be determined.

The major complications following pancreas transplantation are infection, vascular thrombosis, preservation injury, rejection and pancreatitis. Since type I insulin-dependent diabetes mellitus is autoimmune in nature, patients often have autoantibodies in their serum which react with the cytoplasm or surface antigens of the cells of the islets of Langerhans. Histologically, the latter are surrounded by mononuclear cells; the lymphocytes are predominantly CD8 +, thus giving a similar histological picture to that seen in other autoimmune diseases and in graft rejection reactions. Thus, it is difficult to distinguish rejection from autoimmune pathology in patients with transplanted pancreatic tissue. One of the indications of rejection is the loss of control of glucose concentration in the blood. However, this is a relatively late finding and is generally insensitive. The only indicative histological finding is the presence of vasculitis; other abnormal histological findings may be caused by the underlying disease or a reaction to a secondary foreign body associated with the transplantation procedure.

Treatment to prevent rejection is less successful for pancreas than for kidney or liver transplantation. Cyclosporine and corticosteroids are somewhat successful, although a more potent protocol is indicated in patients who have not received a kidney transplant and who are not uraemic. This protocol involves cyclosporine, azathioprine and prednisolone. When evidence of rejection is observed, the patient is treated with intravenous bolus doses of corticosteroids, increased oral prednisolone or a temporary course of anti-lymphocyte globulin.

LUNG AND HEART–LUNG TRANSPLANTATION

Due to the limitations of the technique and supply of donor organs, lung transplantation is still quite rare. Such transplants are indicated in patients with primary pulmonary failure. However, complications arise due to the failure of the bronchial anastomoses to heal. In addition, rejection is diagnosed by changes in respiratory function and by physical changes observable in X-ray images. Current therapy includes the use of cyclosporine, azathioprine and anti-thymocyte globulin in the early post-operative stages and corticosteroids following the initiation of tracheal healing.

LEARNING OUTCOMES

The surgical techniques involved in organ transplantation have improved tremendously in the last 50 years, increasing the life-expectancy of a large number of patients with a wide range of diseases. This chapter has aimed to introduce you to the range of techniques used for transplanting different organs and the complications of the process which may result in rejection. It should have whetted your appetite to learn more about this life-saving therapy and the immunological complications which may be caused by this approach to treatment. The Further Reading contains some relevant literature which will be a good starting point for further studies, and the relevant chapter in the accompanying program should allow you to test your understanding of the subject.

Chapter 16

Immunodeficiency Diseases

LEARNING OBJECTIVES

This chapter concerns those diseases which directly affect the normal functioning of the immune system. Immunodeficiency diseases were first described in the 1950s, when the use of antibiotics and passive immunisation increased the survival of individuals with recurrent infections. Immunodeficiency diseases are characterised by infections caused by organisms which are easily overcome and eliminated in healthy persons. Thus, individuals with immunodeficiency diseases tend to contract infections very easily, have aggressive disease and respond poorly to therapy. The diseases can be broadly segregated into **primary** and **acquired**. Individuals are born with primary immunodeficiency diseases as a result of either **genetic** or **developmental** abnormalities. Acquired immunodeficiencies are those which result from infection or clinical treatment (**iatrogenic immunodeficiency**), e.g. damage to the immune system as a result of radiotherapy for cancer.

In this chapter, we will learn the difference between primary and acquired immunodeficiencies and look at examples of each type of immunodeficiency disease. Although rare, these illnesses serve to illustrate the role of different elements of the immune system in healthy individuals. By looking at the type of infections which occur when a particular part of the immune system is defective, we can gain an insight into those mechanisms which are important in combating specific infectious agents.

CLASSIFICATION OF IMMUNODEFICIENCY DISEASES

Immunodeficiency diseases fall into two principal categories—primary and acquired. The causes of primary immunodeficiency diseases may be **congenital** (due to developmental or genetic abnormalities occurring during pregnancy) or genetic (due to the inheritance of an abnormal gene from one or both parents). Acquired immunodeficiency disease may result from exposure to chemicals, drugs, irradiation or micro-organisms. In recent years, AIDS (the acquired

Table 16.1   Causes of immunodeficiency diseases

Cause	Example
Genetic	Autosomal recessive, autosomal dominant, X-linked, gene deletions and rearrangements
Biochemical and metabolic deficiencies	Adenosine deaminase deficiency
Vitamin or mineral deficiencies	Biotin, zinc
Developmental abnormalities	Cessation of development during embryo-genesis
Autoimmune diseases	Antibodies or T cells with activity towards each other
Acquired immunodeficiency	Viral, transfusion-related, chronic infection, malnutrition, drug abuse, cancer, radiotherapy, chemotherapy, maternal alcoholism

immune deficiency syndrome) has received much attention, but other acquired diseases are becoming more common due to the use of chemo- and radio-therapy. These are known as iatrogenic immunodeficiencies, i.e. acquired as a result of treatment for another clinical condition.

The resulting diseases may be classified according to which part of the immune system is affected, i.e. B cells, T cells, B and T cells, phagocytes, complement or a combination of these.

PRIMARY IMMUNODEFICIENCY DISEASES

Primary immunodeficiency diseases are a diverse group of disorders which arise from a range of genetic abnormalities. Some of these diseases (which may affect one or several parts of the immune system) are extremely rare and the precise underlying defect has not been defined. Examples of each of these diseases will be discussed below.

Table 16.2   Clinical features associated with immunodeficiency

Clinical features
Chronic infection
Unusually frequent, recurrent infection
Failure to completely clear infection
Poor response to treatment
Skin rash
Diarrhoea
Stunted growth
Recurrent abscesses
Recurrent osteomyelitis
Signs and symptoms of autoimmune disease

B Cell Abnormalities

Immunoglobulin A Deficiency

IgA deficiency is the most common of the primary immunodeficiency diseases. Clinically it presents as a heterogeneous group of disorders which include diseases affecting the gastrointestinal tract, allergic reactions, a diverse range of infections, and diseases which are autoimmune or genetic in origin. The clinical presentation of IgA deficiency is dependent upon the degree of abnormal B cell differentiation, the characteristic defect seen in classical IgA deficiency. This arrest in B cell development is thought to be due to **abnormal immunoregulatory signals**, since in patients with this disease the genes coding for immunoglobulin molecules appear to be normal, as does their expression.

IgA-producing B cells have undergone **somatic rearrangement** such that the switch region immediately before the μ gene is joined to the one preceding the α gene and the sequences in between are removed. This process appears to be controlled by transforming growth factor-beta 1 (TGFβ_1). Patients with IgA deficiency appear to have a decrease in the recombination event (when compared with normal individuals), which may be due to the defective production of TGFβ_1. However, the levels of mRNA coding for this cytokine in peripheral blood mononuclear cells isolated from patients with IgA deficiency have been shown to be the same as those in control subjects.

Recently, genetic studies have suggested that the disease is related to the presence of a susceptibility gene in or near the major histocompatibility gene complex which may predispose homozygous individuals to a wide range of antibody deficiencies, from reduced IgA production alone to **panhypogammaglobulinaemia** (reduced levels of all gamma-globulins).

Infantile X-linked Agammaglobulinaemia (XLA)

Newborn babies are normally unable to produce specific antibodies when exposed to an antigen. At this stage, a baby is protected by maternal antibodies which have crossed the placenta. Later (7–9 months of age), normal babies begin to produce their own antibodies. Babies with infantile X-linked agammaglobulinaemia (XLA) are unable to do so and present with recurrent bacterial infections. Individuals affected by this disease (the majority of whom are male) usually have less than 10% of the normal level of serum IgG and less than 1% of the normal serum levels of IgA and IgM. Additionally, they have low levels of B cells and plasma cells. T cells in affected individuals seem to be normal. Thus, as might be expected, viral infections (which are largely controlled by T cells) are rarely life-threatening in patients with XLA.

As the name of the disease suggests, it is genetically based and the defect is inherited from the mother. All cells have a set of paired chromosomes, one half of each pair being maternal, and the other paternal, in origin. In any cell, only one chromosome in each pair is active. In normal women, the active X chromosomes are derived equally from the mother and father. By contrast, in female carriers of a number of X-linked immunodeficiency disorders (including X-linked agammaglobulinaemia, X-linked severe combined immunodeficiency disease, and the Wiskott–Aldrich syndrome) the active X chromosomes are those which carry the abnormal copy of the gene (**allele**).

Several studies suggest that the genetic defect in XLA affects B cell development at a number of different stages (Table 16.3). In addition, recent studies have identified a new cytoplasmic protein, **Bruton's tyrosine kinase (Btk)**, which is mutated in XLA. Since several studies have shown that such cytoplasmic kinases are essential for cell growth and differentiation and are involved in lymphocyte signal transduction, this mutated protein is likely to be involved in the developmental abnormalities seen in XLA. Indeed, the gene coding for Btk maps to the position (**locus**) q22 on the X chromosome, which has been identified as that involved in XLA. In addition, Btk is expressed in B but not T cells, which may explain why, despite the obvious B cell defect in these patients, T cells appear to be functionally and phenotypically normal. Interestingly, the abnormal gene is also expressed in the myeloid cells of patients with XLA. However, these cells appear functionally normal.

T Cell Abnormalities

There are a number of known primary T cell immunodeficiency syndromes which include severe combined immunodeficiency syndrome, Di George syndrome, Wiskott–Aldrich syndrome, ataxia telangiectasia, defective expression of MHC Class II molecules, and defective expression of the CD3–TCR complex. The underlying defects for all these diseases vary, but the principal cell affected in all of them is the T cell. We shall examine Di George syndrome as an example of a typical T cell-related immunodeficiency disorder.

Congenital Thymic Aplasia (Di George syndrome)

In contrast to many other immunodeficiency diseases, which become apparent after the loss of maternal antibodies, Di George syndrome is associated with

Table 16.3   B cell abnormalities reported to be associated with XLA

B cell developmental abnormalities
Reduced pre-B cell proliferation, with fewer cells entering the S-phase of the cell cycle
Failure of pre-B cell to thrive
Inversion of bone marrow ratio of pro- and pre-B cells
Few, immature circulating B cells

symptoms which appear immediately after birth owing to defective T cell function. Affected babies have a range of abnormal clinical features (Table 16.4) and at birth will be **lymphopaenic** (i.e. will have severely decreased numbers of lymphocytes) with very few circulating T cells. In addition, lymphocytes fail to proliferate in response to stimulation with mitogens (e.g. phytohaemagglutinin — PHA) or allogeneic cells. Thus, individuals with this disease must not be immunised with live, attenuated, viral vaccines due to the need for effective cell-mediated immunity to eliminate these organisms. Interestingly, the T cell defect in Di George syndrome may vary from reduced levels of functionally normal T cells to a complete lack of T cell immunity. This variability is probably related to the abnormal thymic development during the first trimester (0–12 weeks) of pregnancy which is associated with this disease.

Although the primary defect in Di George syndrome is T cell-dependent, some patients have low immunoglobulin levels and fail to make specific antibody following immunisation.

T and B Cell Abnormalities

Severe Combined Immunodeficiency Disease (SCID)

Individuals with severe combined immunodeficiency disease (SCID) have defective T and B cell function which prevents the development of normal cell-mediated or humoral responses. One of the features of this disease is a lymphopaenia (severely reduced numbers of circulating lymphocytes) which is largely due to the extremely low number of T cells in the peripheral blood which may fail to express MHC gene products (see the section on **Bare lymphocyte syndrome**). In addition, affected individuals generally have very low serum levels of all classes of immunoglobulin and fail to produce specific antibodies following immunisation or infection.

Due to the T cell abnormality, shortly after birth affected babies may develop disseminated yeast infections (usually caused by *Monilia* spp.), severe pneumonia (caused by *Pneumocystis carinii*) and recurrent infections caused

Table 16.4   Clinical features associated with Di George syndrome

Clinical feature
Low-set ears with notched lobes
A fish-shaped mouth
Slanting eyes
Reduced parathyroid activity (hypoparathyroidism)
Congenital heart disease
Abnormalities of the thymus
Severely impaired cellular immunity

by other opportunistic pathogens (organisms which, in healthy individuals, are normally prevented from causing disease by the immune system). Since these infections usually affect the skin, the pulmonary tract and the gastrointestinal tract, their prevalence in patients with SCID suggests that the defect also affects the immune mechanisms normally involved in surface and mucosal immunity. Since both the cell-mediated and humoral systems are affected, patients may die as a result of infection with common viruses such as varicella, herpes and cytomegalovirus. In addition, affected children often have chronic diarrhoea and malabsorption of nutrients from the gut, resulting in a failure to thrive.

The disease is inherited as an autosomal or X-linked, recessive trait but the genetically determined biochemical defect is unknown for most cases. However, approximately 25% of SCID patients have a deficiency in the **adenosine deaminase (ADA)** enzyme.

SCID with adenosine deaminase deficiency (ADA-SCID). ADA-SCID is inherited as an autosomal, recessive trait. The severe immune deficiency characteristic of this condition is thought to be a direct consequence of the deficiency of the enzyme ADA, which catalyses the conversion of adenosine (Ado) and deoxyadenosine (dAdo) to inosine and deoxyinosine, respectively. In ADA-deficient individuals, dAdo accumulates intracellularly (as well as extracellularly) and becomes phosphorylated to dATP, a compound which is thought to be toxic and is normally not detected at high levels in mammalian cells. Although ADA is normally present in all cells of the body, its absence presents as a defect which characteristically affects the cells of the immune system alone. Individuals with ADA-SCID show severe depletion of T cells in all lymphoid organs and in the peripheral blood. This is thought to be due to the fact that T cells have the greatest concentration of the enzymes which phosphorylate dAdo to dATP and are thus most likely to be killed due to the high intracellular levels of dATP formed. Some B cell abnormalities have been reported to be associated with this condition, but these may result from a lack of normal T cell help rather than from any intrinsic defect.

X-linked, severe combined immunodeficiency (X-SCID). X-SCID is characterised by severely impaired immune responses. Patients lack T cells in their peripheral blood and the B cells which are present are functionally abnormal. Recently, the gene for the γ chain of the interleukin-2 receptor (IL-2R) has been mapped to the same region as the genetic locus associated with X-SCID, i.e. Xq13. From this finding it has been inferred that the defects seen in X-SCID result from abnormal IL-2 function. However, it is not immediately obvious how such a defect might result in the profound immunodeficiency associated with X-SCID. As we discussed earlier, it is common in X-linked immunodeficiencies to see restricted X chromosome activation. Studies of X-SCID female carriers have shown that T cells did not reach maturity if they were carrying the defective IL-2R γ chain gene on the active X chromosome, indicating a role for this gene in normal T cell development. Also, although patients with X-SCID show the same clinical signs and symptoms as those with IL-2 deficiency, the latter group show normal levels of peripheral blood T cells and their defect can be corrected by the addition of exogenous IL-2. This is not so for patients with X-SCID. This therefore presents a paradox, since it might be expected that defective production of either a growth factor or its receptor would have similar consequences. However, the defect in X-SCID is more severe than that in IL-2 deficiency, and this led to the suggestion that the IL-2R γ chain is shared by more than one cytokine receptor; this has subsequently been shown to be the case. The IL-2R γ chain also forms part of the receptors for IL-4 and IL-7, and in all cases is associated with increased receptor-cytokine affinity. It is essential for the internalisation of the IL-7–IL-7R complex, for cellular proliferation stimulated by both IL-4 and IL-7 and for the phosphorylation of a cellular substrate by a tyrosine kinase, an event involved in the internal signalling leading to cellular proliferation and/or differentiation.

Studies on the effect of anti-IL-7 antibodies on the development of T cells in mice suggest that in humans with X-SCID the defective IL-7 receptor-associated γ chain may be responsible for the observed T cell abnormalities. However, one must exercise caution in making direct extrapolations from animal studies, since the treated mice also showed an inhibition of B cell differentiation, a defect not seen in humans with X-SCID. This illustrates the need for further studies to understand the precise role of the γ chain in this disease.

The Bare Lymphocyte Syndrome

Bare lymphocyte syndrome is a rare, primary immunodeficiency disease in which leukocytes fail to express MHC Class II antigens and show defective expression of MHC Class I antigens. As a consequence, affected individuals fail to mount an immune response to foreign antigens.

Symptoms start during the first year of life and affected individuals suffer from recurrent chest infections and chronic diarrhoea. The lack of T cell immunity means that patients may suffer from a range of viral infections (including meningitis and hepatitis) and autoimmune phenomena. Affected individuals do not have a great life-expectancy — the mean age at death in one survey was 4 years, with the main cause of death being viral infection. Recently, treatment by bone marrow transplantation has greatly improved the chances of long-term survival, success being affected by the presence of pre-existing viral infections.

Abnormalities Associated with Phagocytic Cells

Chediak–Higashi Syndrome (CHS)

This is a rare disease arising from an autosomal recessive trait mainly affecting neutrophils. Affected individuals suffer from recurrent, pyogenic infections and have moderately reduced levels of circulating neutrophils (**neutropaenia**) which contain characteristic giant lysosomes. These organelles contain enzymes and other constituents which are usually segregated in distinct cytoplasmic granules.

Chronic Granulomatous Disease (CGD)

Several hundred cases of chronic granulomatous disease (CGD) have been reported since it was first described in the 1950s. Affected individuals present with a variety of clinical features but all have a defect in the oxidative metabolism of phagocytic cells (i.e. neutrophils, monocytes, macrophages and eosinophils). In addition, patients suffer from a great variety of infections caused by bacteria and fungi, and a range of other complications, including **chronic granulomatous inflammation**.

Patients with the classic form of CGD develop serious infections usually within the first year of life. In most cases, infection is caused by *Staphylococcus aureus* and Gram-negative bacilli. However, infection with the fungi *Aspergillus* sp. and *Candida* sp. is also seen. Although severe, infection in CGD may be characterised initially only by malaise, low-grade fever and a mild leukocytosis (raised white cell count) or elevation in erythrocyte sedimentation rate. Organisms which produce H_2O_2 but are catalase negative (e.g. *Streptococcus* sp., *Pneumococcus* sp., *Lactobacillus* sp.) are not major pathogens in CGD. This may be because the H_2O_2 produced by the microbes within the phagosome interacts with the host cell myeloperoxidase (MPO), resulting in bactericidal activity. Alternatively, O_2-independent microbicidal mechanisms may be sufficient in CGD to kill certain pathogens. A diagnosis of CGD is easily confirmed by the **nitroblue tetrazolium reduction test** or other tests of neutrophil oxidative metabolism.

The precise defect in CGD responsible for the decreased microbicidal activity of phagocytic cells has not been fully established. It has been proposed that the electron transport chain involved in oxidative metabolism pumps electrons but not protons into the phagocytic vacuole, leading to pH elevation. This alkalinisation fully activates neutral proteases, which kill bacteria. Thus, an abnormal transport chain in patients with CGD would prevent this outcome. Indeed, a defect in NADPH oxidase has been demonstrated in patients with CGD. Abnormalities in the cytochromes involved in the electron transport chain have also been demonstrated. Nearly all males with X-linked CGD either lack, or have a very abnormal, cytochrome b_{558}. In female carriers, the concentration of this cytochrome correlates directly with the proportion of cells demonstrating inactivation of the abnormal X chromosome. By contrast, about 15% of cases of CGD show an autosomal recessive pattern of transmission; the vast majority of such patients have normal levels of cytochrome b_{558}. It has been suggested that a structural gene for the cytochrome is located on an autosomal chromosome, whilst the X chromosome encodes a putative b cytochrome gene activator, an 'enhancer element' required for appropriate transcription, or a protein (possibly a component of the oxidase) necessary for normal insertion of the cytochrome in the oxidase chain. The complexity of the disease is further shown by the demonstration of reduced flavine adenine dinucleotide (FAD) in CGD neutrophils and selective defects in activation of the respiratory burst by particulate but not soluble stimuli or vice versa.

A further consequence of the abnormal oxidative metabolism associated with CGD is that patients are predisposed to granuloma formation, occasionally resulting in throat, bowel or urogenital tract obstruction. Normal neutrophils inactivate chemoattractants through the **myeloperoxidase–hydrogen peroxide– halide system**. The defect in oxidative metabolism in CGD leads to a lack of H_2O_2 production and thus a failure to inactivate chemoattractants. This is likely to lead to prolonged leukocyte recruitment. In addition, inefficient degradation of antigen may result in the chronic release of cytokines such as interferon-gamma (IFNγ), which may stimulate the granulomatous process.

Abnormalities of the Complement Pathway

Deficiencies of Complement Components

Immunodeficiencies associated with defective complement activity generally behave as autosomal recessive traits. Affected individuals lack, or have reduced levels of, complement proteins, as a result of an abnormal gene. In heterozygous individuals (with one normal and one abnormal gene), reduced protein production occurs. However, since normal serum complement component concentrations vary greatly, it may not be possible to identify those individuals carrying an abnormal gene.

The alternative pathway. The alternative complement pathway is the immediate defence against microbial infection which allows time for specific immunity to develop. Defects in this pathway may result in serious infection, and affected individuals have frequent, severe infections caused by organisms such as *Pneumococcus* spp., *Haemophilus influenzae* and *Staphylococcus* spp.

The classical pathway. Genetic abnormalities which affect the pre-C3 convertase part of the classical complement pathway are not associated with repeated infections, due to the activity of the alternative pathway. In contrast to this, deficiency of C3, which is common to both the classical and alternative pathways, results in severe, potentially fatal infections.

Deficiencies which involve C5 and subsequent complement components do not affect the patient's ability to control most infections, since the opsonic and chemotactic activities of the earlier components are intact. However, individuals with such defects may suffer from repeated infections caused by *Neisseria* spp. and *Meningococcus* spp.; obviously, the lytic activity of the membrane attack complex is needed to eliminate these encapsulated organisms. However, defective C9 is not associated with uncontrollable infection. This is probably because the C5–C8 complex destabilises the membrane enough to mediate lysis of most infectious agents.

Hereditary Angioneurotic Oedema (HANE)

First described in the 1880s, hereditary angioneurotic oedema (HANE) is an autosomal dominant disease which results from the lack of a protein which inhibits the action of the first component of complement (**C1INH**).This protease inhibitor is also involved in the regulation of the coagulation, fibrinolytic and contact (or kinin-forming) systems. Lack of C1 inhibitor results in a range of severe symptoms (Table 16.5) and biochemical defects, reflecting the importance of this protein.

Biochemically, the decreased level of C1 inhibitor leads to low serum levels of C2 and C4 due to the uncontrolled activation of C1. The central role played by C1 inhibitor in the control of the complement, clotting and kinin systems means that, after an appropriate stimulus (trauma or stress), affected individuals undergo a massive inflammatory response. The implications of this may be seen in patients who have an oedematous reaction in their larynx. The swelling blocks the airway and, unless treated immediately, the patient will die. In order to prevent such attacks, patients are treated with long-term androgen therapy. It is thought that this hormone may enhance the synthesis of C1 inhibitor by the liver.

Hereditary angioneurotic oedema is classified as either Type I or Type II. Patients with Type I HANE (85% of affected individuals) have very low levels of C1 inhibitor (5–30% of normal plasma levels). In contrast to this, patients

Table 16.5 Clinical characteristics of hereditary angioneurotic oedema

Clinical characteristics
Episodic, acute local oedema of the skin or mucosa affecting mainly the extremities, face, larynx and gut
Attacks (which are often associated with trauma or emotional stress) last from 24 to 72 hours
Attacks begin in childhood and increase in severity during adolescence
Frequency and severity of attacks decreases by the fifth or sixth decade of life. Also in pregnant women, particularly in the second and third trimesters

with Type II HANE have normal or elevated levels of C1 inhibitor. However, a large proportion of this protein is dysfunctional; only a very low level of the normal protein is present. It has been suggested that the two forms of the disease result from different genetic abnormalities. Type I HANE is thought to be due to a defect in a regulator gene, whilst patients with Type II HANE most probably have a structural gene defect.

ACQUIRED IMMUNODEFICIENCIES

Iatrogenic Immunodeficiencies

Iatrogenic immunodeficiencies are a consequence of our advances in patient care and therapy. They are a heterogeneous group of immunodeficiency diseases, the limits of which are difficult to delineate. However, they are all induced by the use of treatment regimes which result in temporary or permanent immunodeficiency (Table 16.6).

The incidence of iatrogenic immunodeficiencies is rapidly increasing as a consequence of the increase in chemotherapeutic treatment for cancer and leukaemia and the more widespread use of organ and bone marrow transplantation for treatment of terminal illnesses.

Since this form of acquired immunodeficiency results from therapeutic regimes, its occurrence depends upon the strength and/or duration of the therapy. However, presentation and outcome of the disease may also be affected by other factors (Table 16.7).

The Acquired Immunodeficiency Syndrome (AIDS)

AIDS probably has become the most widely publicised infectious disease and, in the years since its first description, has been the subject of a mountain of both

Table 16.6 Causes of iatrogenic immunodeficiency disease

Treatment	Treatment for
X- or gamma-irradiation	Cancer, leukaemia and immunologically mediated diseases
Corticosteroids or other immunosuppressive drugs	Cancer, leukaemia and immunologically mediated diseases; transplantation
Antibiotics	Infection; may indirectly cause proliferation of potentially harmful bacteria or fungi by altering the intestinal flora of the host; part of the innate immune system
Gold salts or other chemo-therapeutic agents	Autoimmune diseases; may cause alterations in the haemopoietic system, producing anaemia, granulocyto-paenia, thrombocytopaenia or immune deficiency

Table 16.7 Factors affecting the presentation and outcome of iatrogenic immuno-deficiencies

Factors affecting presentation of disease	Example
The type of disease for which treatment is being given	Treatment of autoimmune diseases may lead to immunodeficiency
Reactivation of latent infections in the host	Treatment may eliminate immunoregulatory mechanisms which keep infections in check, resulting in overwhelming and life-threatening infections
Allogeneic stimulation	Patients receiving blood transfusions or organ transplants who are therapeutically immunosuppressed may suffer from graft-versus-host disease caused by the immunologically active cells in the grafts
Exposure to infectious agents after development of immunodeficiency	Immunocompromised hosts are not able to fight off even common infections

scientific and popular literature. It is not possible in a book like this to fully describe the extent of our knowledge of AIDS and its causative virus — the **human immunodeficiency virus** (HIV). The vast amount of research being performed in this area means that this section could be out of date before the book is published. Thus, it is my aim to introduce the topic at a fundamental level; publications in the Further Reading cover in more depth the recent advances concerning the disease and virus.

AIDS was first identified as a result of a study at the Centers for Disease Control in Atlanta, Georgia. It was noticed that a number of otherwise apparently healthy young men had died of opportunistic infections which normally only kill individuals with some underlying, predisposing immunodeficiency. The types of infections which killed these individuals and were found to be affecting others like them would normally be controlled by cell-mediated immune mechanisms. Thus, further studies of affected individuals concentrated on examining their peripheral blood lymphocytes. These showed that the patients had decreased levels of circulating CD4+ T cells. This led to a search for a causative agent which might be infecting and destroying T cells. This resulted in the identification of a virus which eventually became known as the human immunodeficiency virus or HIV.

The Human Immunodeficiency Virus (HIV)

HIV has been classified as a lentivirus, due to its cone-shaped core which contains the viral genetic code (ribonucleic acid — RNA) and an enzyme which allows the transcription of this viral RNA into deoxyribonucleic acid (DNA).

The core is surrounded by an envelope which consists of knobs made up of trimers or tetramers of the envelope glycoproteins (Figure 16.1). These glycoproteins are derived from a precursor molecule gp160, which is cleaved inside the cell to give the gp120 and gp41 proteins. The gp120 glycoprotein contains the virus receptor for cellular binding and the major neutralising sites. The gp41 protein plays an important role in virus–cell and cell–cell fusion.

The genome of HIV is about 9.8 kb long and the primary transcript produces a messenger RNA which is translated into the Gag and Pol proteins (Figure 16.2). The Gag proteins (p25, p17, p9 and p6) are derived from a precursor molecule, p55, and form the capsid (p25), the nucleocapsid (p17) and the core (p17) proteins of the virus. The Pol proteins derived from the Pol precursor molecule include the protease responsible for cleaving precursor proteins, the integrase involved in viral integration into the host cell genome and the reverse transcriptase (or RNA-dependent DNA polymerase) which converts the viral RNA genome into DNA. In addition to these products, others are produced as a result of splicing mRNA. These include the product of the *rev* gene (itself the result of mRNA splicing) which regulates the relative production of unspliced, singly or multiply spliced mRNAs. Other products of multiply spliced mRNA include a range of regulatory and accessory proteins which control virus production (Table 16.8).

Attachment of HIV of the host cell is via the CD4 which is expressed on a subset of T cells and on some monocytes/macrophages. Binding to CD4 is

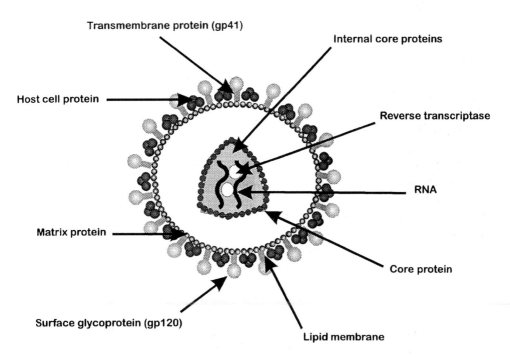

Figure 16.1 Structure of the human immunodeficiency virus

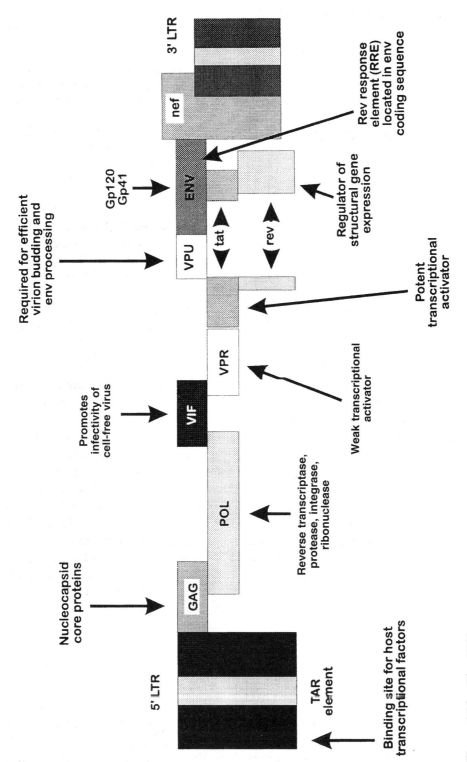

Figure 16.2 The HIV genome

Table 16.8   Regulatory proteins of HIV

Gene product	Effect
Tat (transactivating protein)	Binds the TAR (Tat responsive region) in the 3′ portion of the viral long terminal repeat region (LTR) and is the main HIV replication-enhancing protein
Rev (Regulator of viral expression)	Binds the Rev-responsive element in the viral envelope mRNA and permits unspliced mRNA to leave the nucleus and enter the cytoplasm, thus allowing the production of full-length viral proteins which are needed for infectious virus production
Nef (Negative factor)	Has a variety of functions, including down-regulation of viral expression. It may cause this effect by interacting with the viral LTR or by interfering with Rev binding to the envelope mRNA
Vif, Vpr, Vpu/Vpx (accessory proteins)	These proteins are important in virus assembly and budding and in the infectivity and production of infectious virus

thought to cause conformational changes in gp120 which, along with cleavage of the envelope protein by cellular enzymes, cause another change in the viral envelope, leading to virus–cell fusion.

Once the virus has entered the cell, a sequence of events occurs which results in the integration of the provirus into the host genome (Figure 16.3). The virus genome is reverse transcribed by the viral RNA-dependent DNA polymerase, giving rise to a double-stranded DNA provirus which migrates to the nucleus of the cell and randomly integrates into the host genome. Replication of the virus appears to depend to some degree on the activation state and nature of the infected cells. T lymphocytes in the G_0 stage of the cell cycle undergo abortive infection, whilst non-dividing macrophages are able to produce infectious virus. By contrast, T cells activated by antigen and a variety of lymphokines are permissive to virus infection, HIV undergoing integration and replication within approximately 24 hours (Figure 16.4).

Consequences of HIV Infection

As a result of HIV infection, patients present with a number of immunological abnormalities affecting both B and T cell function. Antibody levels are typically elevated due to polyclonal activation of B cells, but patients show an inability to respond to antigens to which they have been previously exposed. The most notable abnormality in these individuals is the gradual loss of CD4+ cells.

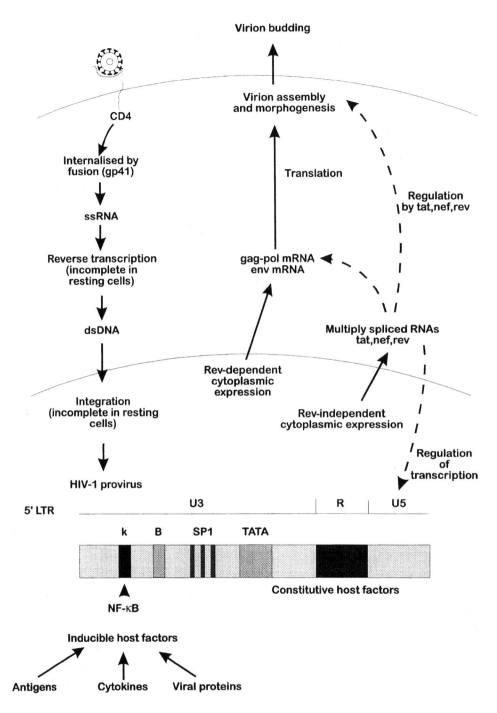

Figure 16.3   Mechanisms involved in HIV replication

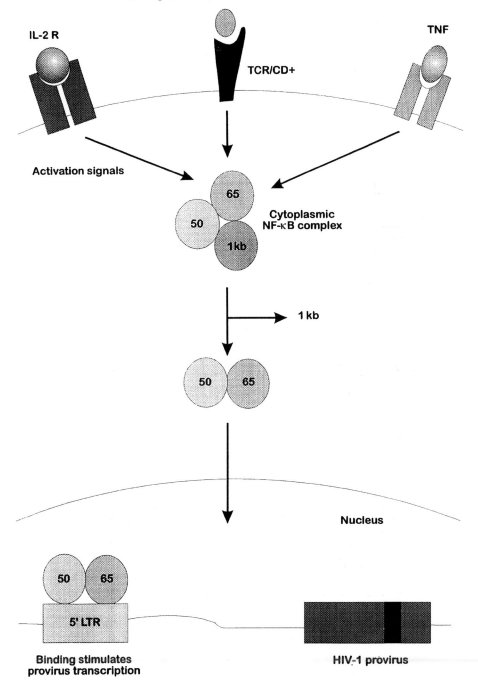

Figure 16.4   Mechanisms involved in cellular activation leading to HIV transcription

Table 16.9   The principal opportunistic infections and tumours in HIV infection

Classification	Opportunistic agent
Bacteria	*Mycobacteria avium intracellulare*
	Mycobacterium tuberculosis
	Salmonella spp.
Viruses	Cytomegalovirus
	Varicella zoster
	Herpes simplex
Fungi	*Pneumocystis carinii*
	Cryptococcus neoformans
	Candida
Parasites	*Toxoplasma* spp.
	Cryptosporidium spp.
	Leishmania spp.
Malignancies	Kaposi's sarcoma
	Burkitt's lymphoma

There are many explanations for the severe loss of CD4+ cells, which cannot merely be the result of the destruction of the cells as a result of virus replication. These abnormalities severely affect the ability of the individual to respond to infection, resulting in overwhelming infections from which the patients die. Some of the opportunistic infections and tumours which become life-threatening in the terminal stages of AIDS are listed in Table 16.9.

LEARNING OUTCOMES

This chapter has introduced you to a range of very different diseases which all have an underlying abnormality resulting in a defect in the immune system. All the patients are likely to succumb sooner or later to life-threatening infections. You should now understand the difference between primary and acquired immunodeficiency diseases. The former are relatively rare, whilst the latter are showing increased incidences. It is important that you understand how HIV may be acquired and the way in which it causes disease, and to this end you should read some of the excellent articles listed in the Further Reading. In addition, this chapter should have made you appreciate the way in which clinical signs and symptoms may give us clues about the underlying abnormalities present in a patient and how abnormalities which affect certain elements of the immune system may allow us to gain a greater understanding of the working of the normal immune system.

References

Aspinall RL, Meyer RK, Graetzer MA, Wolfe HR (1963) Effect of thymectomy and bursectomy on the survival of skin homografts in chickens. *J Immunol* **90**: 872.

Bach JF, Dormont J, Dardenne M, Balner H (1969) In vitro rosette inhibition by anti-human anti-lymphocyte serum. Correlation with skin graft prolongation in subhuman primates. *Transplantation* **8**: 265.

Glick B, Chang TG, Joap RG (1956) The bursa of Fabricius and antibody production. *Poultry Sci* **35**: 224.

Ohashi PS, Mak TW, Vandenelsen P, Yanagi Y, Yoshikai Y, Calman AF, Terhorst C, Stobo JD, Weiss A (1985) Reconstitution of an active surface T3 T-cell antigen receptor by DNA transfer. *Nature* **316**: 606.

Tiselius A, Kabat EA (1939) An electrophoretic study of immune sera and purified antibody preparations. *J Exp Med* **69**: 119.

Further Reading

CHAPTER 1

Austyn JM (1989) *Antigen-presenting cells.* In Focus series (eds D Rickwood and D Male). IRL Press at OUP, Oxford.

■ The 'In Focus' series were a group of relatively brief publications covering particular topics. Although they are now rather old (rumour has it that new editions are being considered), they provide an excellent introduction to the topics they cover. You should also read the book in the series which is called *Complement* as an accompaniment to Chapter 5.

Cosman D (1989) Colony-stimulating factors in vivo and in vitro. *Immunol Today* **9**: 97–98.

■ This brief review describes the nature and activity of colony-stimulating factors.

Graham GJ, Pragnell IB (1992) The haemopoietic stem cell: properties and control mechanisms. *Semin Cell Biol* **3**: 423–434.

■ This provides a detailed description of the properties of the haemopoietic stem cell and the factors which regulate its proliferation and differentiation.

Klaus GGB (1990) *B Lymphocytes.* IRL Press at OUP, Oxford.

■ This is another in the 'In Focus' series which, although a little old now, covers the basics of B cell biology very well. Much of the content is relevant to other chapters in this book.

Ritter MA, Crispe IN (1992) *The Thymus.* IRL Press at OUP, Oxford.

■ This excellent little book in the 'In Focus' series, published in association with the British Society for Immunology, gives a comprehensive account of the structure, function, development and population dynamics of the thymus. Whilst the volume of information it contains may be too great for the new student, it is eminently readable. Although the terminology may be confusing at times, the book contains a concise glossary to help with the ever-present acronyms.

Smith SP, Yee GC (1992) Hematopoiesis. *Pharmacotherapy* **12**(2pt2): 11S–19S.

■ This article covers the basics of haematopoiesis, describing the environment (bone marrow) in which it takes place and the cells which constitute the circulatory system. It gives a basic description of the cells which derive from the stem cell and the cytokines which stimulate their production.

Sprent J, Tough DF (1994) Lymphocyte life-span and memory. *Science* **265**: 1395–1400.
This article describes the development of T and B cells in the primary lymphoid tissues and the development of memory. It also discusses the implications of this development for vaccination. It is relatively easy to read but I would recommend you come back to it at a later stage after studying the chapters on adaptive immunity and tolerance.

Steinman RM (1991) The dendritic cell system and its role in immunogenicity. *Annu Rev Immunol* **9**: 271–296.
This is a comprehensive review of the dendritic cell system which describes their phenotype, differentiation and unique function. It is informative and eminently readable.

Zipori D (1992) The renewal and differentiation of hemopoietic stem cells. *FASEB J* **6**: 2691–2697.
This article describes the organisation of the stem cells, and the control of their differentiation and proliferation. It explains the need for control and the role of cytokines in this process.

CHAPTER 2

Arnon R, Van Regenmortel MHV (1992) Structural basis of antigenic specificity and design of new vaccines. *FASEB J* **6**: 3265–3274.
This review discusses approaches to identifying antigenic epitopes and the factors affecting the immunogenicity of peptides. This is an interesting article and demonstrates the need for an understanding of fundamental immunology before attempting manipulation of the immune system by vaccines or immunomodulatory therapy. However, I recommend that you read this article after studying the chapters on adaptive immunity and tolerance.

Cresswell P (1994) Assembly, transport and function of MHC Class II molecules. *Annu Rev Immunol* **12**: 259–293.
This detailed review article describes the structure of the MHC Class II molecules and the way in which they are assembled, associate with processed peptide and are presented at the cell surface. It is a very good, informative review.

Engelhard VH (1994) Structure of peptides associated with class I and class II MHC molecules. *Annu Rev Immunol* **12**: 181–207.
This article presents a review of the structure of MHC molecules and looks at the peptide molecules that are found naturally associated with them.

Hood L, Steinmetz M, Malissen B (1983) Genes of the Major Histocompatibility Complex of the mouse. *Annu Rev Immunol* **1**: 529–568.
This is a rather old but extensive article which examines the genes of the murine MHC.

Lafuse WP (1991) Molecular biology of murine MHC class II genes. *Crit Rev Immunol* **11**: 167–194.
■ This describes the molecular approach to murine MHC immune response genes. It is quite a complex review but one which reviews the organisation and function of the Ia genes.

Sadegh-Nasseri S, Germain RN (1992) How MHC class II molecules work: peptide-dependent completion of protein folding. *Immunol Today* **13**: 43–46.
■ This review discusses the experimental work which has led to the suggestion that peptide confers a stable structure on the MHC Class II dimer, resulting in a long-lived stable MHC–peptide dimer.

CHAPTER 3

Bentley GA, Boulot G, Karjalainen K, Mariuzza RA (1995) Crystal structure of the b chain of a T cell antigen receptor. *Science* **267**: 1984–1987.

Borst H, Brouns GS, de Vries E, Verschuren MCM, Mason DY, van Dongen JJM (1993) Antigen receptors on T and B lymphocytes: parallels in organisation and functions. *Immunol Rev* **132**: 49–84.
■ This provides a detailed comparison of the structure of the T and B cell antigen–receptor complexes. It is an excellent source of relevant references. It is not easy to read as a novice, due to the assumed knowledge. However, for those who persevere, it gives a comprehensive comparison of the two major antigen recognition structures.

Moss PA, Rosenberg WM, Bell JI (1992) The human T cell receptor in health and disease. *Annu Rev Immunol* **10**: 71–96.
■ This is a comprehensive review of the structure of the T cell receptors. The article also looks at the function of these molecules and their role in health and disease.

Spiegelberg HL (1989) Biological role of different antibody classes. *Int Arch Allergy Appl Immunol* **90**: 22–27.
■ This paper give a synopsis of the biological functions of antibody isotypes. The second part of the paper is less informative, since it deals with cytokine control of class switching, which is covered better in other articles mentioned in the Further Reading for Chapter 6.

CHAPTER 4

Harriman W, Volk H, Defranoux N, Wabl M (1993) Immunoglobulin class switch recombination. *Annu Rev Immunol* **11**: 361–384.
■ This review article describes the molecular events that are involved in the generation of antibody diversity. It covers this complex topic very thoroughly but be warned that you may need a science dictionary if your genetics is not up to scratch!

Kaye J, Kersh G, Engel I, Hedrick SM (1991) Structure and specificity of the T cell antigen receptor. *Semin Immunol* **3**: 269–281.
This review briefly describes the physical structure of the T cell antigen receptor and concentrates on the genetic elements which affect the structure of the antigen-binding region of the TCR.

Owen MJ, Lamb JR (1988) *Immune Recognition*. IRL Press at OUP, Oxford.
The 'In Focus' series are a group of short booklets dedicated to a specific topic. They are aimed at a basic level and progress through up-to-date information on the subject. They present the data in a straightforward and clearly understandable manner. The chapters are well structured and referenced.

Purkerson J, Isakson P (1992) A two-signal model for regulation of immunoglobulin isotype switching. *FASEB J* **6**: 3245–3252.
This review describes the molecular events involved in immunoglobulin class switching. It is thoroughly readable and goes on to discuss the need for direct T cell contact in this process and not just the production of cytokines by these cells.

Robey E, Fowlkes BJ (1994) Selective events in T cell development. *Annu Rev Immunol* **12**: 875–705.
This paper describes the development of T cells, including the generation of diversity in the T cell antigen receptor. Some of you may find it difficult, and many references to mouse studies and murine genes may be confusing, but it is a very detailed review with which it is worth persevering.

Schatz DG, Oettinger MA, Schlissel MS (1992) V(D)J recombination: molecular biology and regulation. *Annu Rev Immunol* **10**: 359–383.
This is a good review article comparing the mechanisms involved in the generation of diversity in both antibodies and the T cell receptor. The paper also considers the structure, function and genomic organisation of the recombination activation genes.

Van Dyk L, Meek K (1992) Assembly of IgH CDR3: mechanism, regulation, and influence on antibody diversity. *Int Rev Immunol* **8**: 123–133.
This review describes the '12–23' rule and the way in which it governs the recombination of VD and J genes to generate antibody diversity. It also describes the experimental evidence for the regulation of VDJ recombination. It is quite complex for the novice, but that is difficult to avoid with this particular topic.

CHAPTER 5

Fearon DT, Austen KF (1980) The alternative pathway of complement — a system for host resistance to microbial infection. *N Engl J Med* **303**: 259–263.
This article describes the activation and control of the alternative pathway. It discusses the nature of the relevant effector molecules, which include inhibitors which deactivate components of the pathway. It also describes a number of clinical conditions related to abnormal complement activity.

Hugli TE (1984) Structure and function of the anaphylatoxins. *Springer Semin Immunopathol* **7**: 193–219.

This is an older review which gives great detail concerning the contemporary knowledge of the structure of the anaphylatoxins and their receptors. However, the article does deal quite well with the function of these molecules.

Jose PJ (1987) Complement-derived peptide mediators of inflammation. *Br Med Bull* **43**: 336–349.

This article discusses the role of complement components, particularly C5a and C3a, in inflammation.

Miller MD, Krangel MS (1992) Biology and biochemistry of the chemokines: a family of chemotactic and inflammatory cytokines. *Crit Rev Immunol* **12**:17–46.

This article describes a group of 14 related inflammatory cytokines known as chemokines. These include IL-8, macrophage inflammatory proteins 1a and 1b, monocyte chemoattractant protein and RANTES. These molecules induce the migration and activation of a variety of cells, including neutrophils, monocytes, lymphocytes and fibroblasts, which play a role in inflammation and repair of tissue damage. The structure and function of each of these cytokines is discussed in detail.

Ninnemann JL (1984) Prostaglandin structure and chemistry: a primer. *Immunol Today* **5**: 172–173.

This is a concise article describing the structure and production of prostaglandins. It should be easily understood even by non-biochemists!

Ninnemann JL (1984) Prostaglandins in inflammation and disease. *Immunol Today* **5**: 173–175.

This article follows the one above and is written in the same easy style. It concisely describes the role of prostaglandins in inflammation and their effects on the immune response in disease.

Nusinow SR, Zuraw BL, Curd JG (1985) The hereditary and acquired deficiencies of complement. *Med Clin North Am* **69**: 487–504.

This article gives a brief description of the complement cascade and describes the role of complement in inflammation, and autoimmune and immunodeficiency diseases.

CHAPTER 6

Akira S, Taga T, Kishimoto T (1993) Interleukin-6 in biology and medicine. *Adv Immunol* **54**: 1–77.

This is a long and comprehensive review of the production, regulation and activity of interleukin-6. It is probably rather complex for the beginner—see the review by Wolvekamp and Marquet instead.

Altman A, Coggeshall KM, Mustelin T (1990) Molecular events mediating T cell activation. *Adv Immunol* **48**: 227–360.

■ This is a very extensive review which, although rather old, describes the molecules and pathways involved in the intracellular signals leading to T cell activation. This is complex for the beginner but is very thorough.

Banchereau J, Blanchard D, Briere F, Galizzi J-P, Garrone P, Lebecque S, Rousset F (1993) Role of cytokines in human B lymphocyte growth and differentiation. *Nouv Rev Fr Hematol* **35**: 61–66.
This easily understandable paper describes the stages involved in B lymphocyte differentiation and discusses the role of cytokines and CD40 in the process.

Berke G (1994) The binding and lysis of target cells by cytotoxic lymphocytes: molecular and cellular aspects. *Annu Rev Immunol* **12**: 735–773.
This is a very detailed review article covering all aspects of the cytotoxic mechanisms in T lymphocytes and NK cells. It is particularly good for the description of experimental investigations which led to our understanding of the process of cytolysis. You should read this reference and try to understand the theory and practice behind the experimental techniques employed.

Coffman RL, Savelkoul HFJ, Lebman DA (1989) Cytokine regulation of immunoglobulin isotype switching and expression. *Semin Immunol* **4**: 55–63.
This paper describes the role of cytokines in regulating isotype switching and antibody expression. It is relatively old but easy to read. Thus, although it largely discusses the situation in mice and the human situation is considered only briefly at the end, it is worth reading.

Coffman RL, Lebman DA, Rothman P (1993) Mechanism and regulation of immunoglobulin isotype switching. *Adv Immunol* **54**: 229–270.
This is a complex review describing the events involved in Ig class switching at both the genetic and cellular level. It is not easy to read, due to the constant listing of references in the middle of sentences, but it is comprehensive, with numerous examples of experimental evidence.

Dorken H (1993) Expression of B-cell associated antigens during B-cell ontogeny. *Recent Results Cancer Res* **131**: 9–18.

Farrar JJ, Benjamin WR, Cheng L, Pawson BA (1984) Interleukin 2. *Annu Rep Med Chem* **19**: 191–200.
Although old, this review describes the biology, chemistry and activity of interleukin-2. Although much more is now known about the reactions involved in IL-2 stimulation of T cells, this is easy to follow and a good place to start to build your understanding of the subject.

Farrar MA, Schreiber RD (1993) The molecular cell biology of interferon-γ and its receptor. *Annu Rev Immunol* **11**: 571–611.
This is a well-written, easy-to-read review of the production, activity and regulation of interferon-gamma.

Grabstein KH, Eisenman J, Shanebeck K, Rauch C, Srinivasan S, Fung V, Beers C, Richardson J, Schoenborn MA, Ahdieh M, Johnson L, Alderson MR, Watson JD, Anderson DM, Giri JG (1994) Cloning of a T cell growth factor that interacts with the b chain of the interleukin-2 receptor. *Science* **264**: 965–968.
This paper describes the cloning and characterisation of interleukin-15, a molecule which shares biological properties with IL-2 and uses part of the IL-2 receptor. It describes the complex techniques involved which, if you find confusing, you should read about in a book describing molecular biology or immunology techniques.

Germain RN, Margulies DH (1993) The biochemistry and cell biology of antigen processing and presentation. *Annu Rev Immunol* **11**: 403–450.
  This is a comprehensive review of the structure of MHC Class I and Class II molecules and the methods of generation of the peptides which are presented by them to T cells. It is very detailed but you should find it relatively easy to read and comprehend.

Hodes RJ (1989) T helper cell–B cell interaction: the roles of direct Th–B cell contact and cell-free mediators. *Semin Immunol* **1**: 33–42.
  This review article clearly explains the role of B cells as antigen-presenting cells and the interaction of the two to give T and B cell activation.

Larrick JW, Wright SC (1992) Native cytokine antagonists. *Baillière's Clin Haematol* **5**: 681–702.
  As we have already seen, the immune system is tightly controlled. The effect of cytokines is regulated in many ways, including through the production of antagonists. This review describes those antagonists and their modes of action.

Linsley PS, Ledbetter JA (1993) The role of the CD28 receptor during T cell responses to antigen. *Annu Rev Immunol* **11**: 191–212.
  This review describes the co-stimulatory activity of CD28. It is quite a complex article and its terminology is already rather out of date, due to the rapid developments in this field. However, it does give a good explanation of the role of co-stimulatory molecules and has an extensive bibliography.

Lyons M, Moses HL (1990) Transforming growth factors and the regulation of cell proliferation. *Eur J Biochem* **187**: 467–471.
  This is a brief review describing the structure and function of transforming growth factor-alpha and -beta. It is informative and concise.

Minami Y, Kono Y, Miyazaki T, Taniguchi T (1993) The IL-2 receptor complex: its structure, function and target genes. *Annu Rev Immunol* **11**: 245–267.
  This is a quite complex but comprehensive review article which describes the molecular components of the IL-2 receptor and its related receptors. It also describes the signal transduction pathways associated with IL-2 receptor ligation.

Moore KW, O'Garra A, de Waal Malefyt R, Vierira P, Mosmann TR (1993) Interleukin-10. *Annu Rev Immunol* **11**: 165–190.
  This detailed review describes the activity of interleukin-10, including its role in the regulation of the development of Th1 and Th2 subsets.

Mosmann TR, Coffman RL (1989) Heterogeneity of cytokine secretion patterns and functions of helper T cells. *Adv Immunol* **46**: 111–147.
  This is a detailed review article from the group which originally established the presence of Th1 and Th2 cells in mice. Although it is a little old and lacking some of the up-to-date names for certain cytokines, it is still an informative review concerning the roles and actions of the T cell subsets.

Parker DC (1993) T cell-dependent B cell activation. *Annu Rev Immunol* **11**: 331–360.
  This is a detailed review article describing the molecular and cellular processes involved in T-dependent, B cell activation. It is rather complex but exhaustive — worth a read.

Paul WE, Seder RA (1994) Lymphocyte responses and cytokines. *Cell* **76**: 241–251.
  This article discusses the role of cytokines in governing lymphocyte responses to antigen. It describes the regulation of T helper subset development by cytokines and how T cell-derived cytokines influence antibody responses. It illustrates points by describing experimental work performed by others. It is not easy for the novice to read but is worth the effort.

Purkerson J, Isakson P (1992) A two-signal model for regulation of immunoglobulin isotype switching. *FASEB J* **6**: 3245–3252.
  This is an informative review which describes regulation of isotype switching in mice and humans. It discusses the cytokines involved and their effects and the need for secondary cellular signals.

Scott P (1993) IL-12: initiation cytokine for cell-mediated immunity. *Science* **260**: 496–497.
  This is a brief article describing the role of IL-12 in the development of the Th1 response to antigen and proposing the use of IL-12 in therapy and in vaccine development.

Seder RA, Paul WE (1994) Acquisition of lymphokine-producing phenotype by CD4 + T cells. *Annu Rev Immunol* **12**: 635–673.
  This is another very readable review by these authors, explaining the complex story of cytokine production by Th subsets.

Sprent J (1994) T and B memory cells. *Cell* **76**: 315–322.
  This review describes the development of T and B memory cells and their recirculation. It is well written and generally easy to read.

Vassalli P (1992) The pathophysiology of tumor necrosis factors. *Annu Rev Immunol* **10**: 411–480.
  This is a detailed review of the functions and effects of tumour necrosis factor.

Vitetta ES, Berton MT, Burger C, Kepron M, Lee WT, Yin X-M (1991) Memory B and T cells. *Annu Rev Immunol* **9**: 193–217.
  This article reviews the properties of memory T and B cells and the mechanisms which result in their generation and activation.

Wolvekamp MCJ, Marquet RL (1990) Interleukin-6: historical background, genetics and biological significance. *Immunol Lett* **24**: 1–10.
  This is a brief, straightforward review concerning the production, regulation and activity of interleukin-6.

CHAPTER 7

Durham SR (1993) Allergic inflammation. *Pediatr Allergy Immunol* **4**: S7–S12.
  This review looks at human allergic responses in vivo which suggest that Th2 cytokines regulate both the IgE-dependent events and tissue eosinophilia in allergy.

Frieri M (1992) Systemic sclerosis. The role of the mast cell and cytokines. *Ann Allergy* **69**: 385–392, 395–396.
   This review deals with the pathophysiology of systemic sclerosis. It is a clinically based article and so non-medically trained individuals may find some of the clinical terminology confusing.

Huntley JF (1992) Mast cells and basophils: a review of their heterogeneity and function. *J Comp Pathol* **107**: 349–372.

Leavitt RY, Fauci AS (1991) Wegener's granulomatosis. *Curr Opin Rheumatol* **3**: 8–14.
   This review studies the current publications concerning Wegner's granulomatosis. This is a disease of unknown aetiology typified by the presence of granulomatous vasculitis in the upper and lower respiratory tracts and by glomerulonephritis. Other papers in this issue also look at aspects of the disease and its therapy.

McEwen BJ (1992) Eosinophils: a review. *Vet Res Commun* **16**: 11–44.
   This review of the structure and function of mammalian eosinophils highlights their role in allergic reactions and in anti-parasitic immunity.

Silver MR, Messner LV (1994) Sarcoidosis and its ocular manifestations. *J Am Optom Assoc* **65**: 321–327.
   Sarcoidosis is characterised by a delayed hypersensitivity (type IV) reaction. This review looks at the epidemiology, pathogenesis and clinical features of non-ocular and ocular sarcoidosis.

Tan HP, Lebeck LK, Nehlsen-Cannarella SL (1992) Regulatory role of cytokines in IgE-mediated allergy. *J Leukocyte Biol* **52**: 115–118.
   This article discusses the role of cytokines in regulating the production of IgE, which is pivotal to the allergic response.

Vercelli D (1993) Regulation of IgE synthesis. *Allergy Proc* **14**: 413–416.
   This review looks at the regulation of IgE production in humans in relation to allergic disease.

CHAPTER 8

Crispe N (1988) Mechanisms of self-tolerance. *Immunol Today* **9**: 329–331.
   This report of a meeting on tolerance mechanisms reviews recent (at the time) advances in the understanding of these mechanisms. It provides some information but has no references for follow-up reading.

Cruse JM, Lewis RE Jr (1993) The immune system victorious: selective preservation of self. *Immunol Res* **12**: 101–114.

Hartwig M (1993) Control of clonal deletion in the thymus: implications for tolerance induction. *Immunol Cell Biol* **71**: 337–340.

Houssaint E, Flajnik M (1990) The role of thymic epithelium in the acquisition of tolerance. *Immunol Today* **11**: 357–360.

Jones LA, Chin LT, Kruisbeek AM (1990) Acquisition of self-tolerance in T cells is achieved by different mechanisms, operating both inside and outside the thymus. *Thymus* **16**: 195–206.

Lo D (1992) T-cell tolerance. *Curr Opin Immunol* **4**: 711–715.

Miller JF (1993) Self–nonself discrimination and tolerance in T and B lymphocytes. *Immunol Res* **12**: 115–130.

Nemazee D, Russell D, Arnold B, Haemmerling G, Allison J, Miller JF, Morahan G, Buerki K (1991) Clonal deletion of autospecific B lymphocytes. *Immunol Rev* **122**: 117–132.

Nossal GJV (1994) Negative selection of lymphocytes. *Cell* **76**: 229–239.
■ This is a very readable paper describing the different methods of tolerance induction in both T cells and B cells. It is worth reading, especially if you find the concept of tolerance difficult to grasp.

StCSinclair NR, Panoskaltsis A (1988) The immunoregulatory apparatus and autoimmunity. *Immunol Today* **9**: 260–265.
■ This is a review which discusses the role of antigen distribution in the development of tolerance. It is easy to read.

CHAPTER 9

Esch T, Clark L, Zhang XM, Goldman S, Heber-Katz E (1992) Observations, legends, and conjectures concerning restricted T-cell receptor usage and autoimmune disease. *Crit Rev Immunol* **11**: 249–264.
■ Several studies have suggested that the repertoire of T cell antigen receptor genes used in autoimmune diseases is highly restricted. This has important implications concerning the recognition of self-antigens and the pathology seen in many autoimmune diseases. Molecular studies such as these are very important, because it is at this fundamental level that the breakdown of self-tolerance occurs, resulting in the complex pathology of these diseases.

Martin R, McFarland HF, McFarlin DE (1992) Immunological aspects of demyelinating diseases. *Annu Rev Immunol* **10**: 153–187.
■ This is a review describing the factors which influence immunological reactions in patients with the autoimmune disease multiple sclerosis. It also makes a comparison with the experimental animal disease allergic encephalomyelitis, which shares some pathological features with MS.

Opdenakker G, van Damme J (1994) Cytokine-regulated proteases in autoimmune diseases. *Immunol Today* **15**: 103–107.
■ This article considers the so-called REGA model of autoimmunity in which non-specific immune mechanisms result in the initiation of autoimmune disease. It looks at the importance of cytokines and proteinases in the initiation of multiple sclerosis and relates these observations to other autoimmune diseases. This is a clearly written article which offers a perspective on the relevance of specific immune responses in the onset of autoimmunity.

Protti MP, Manfredi AA, Horton RM, Bellone M, Conti-Tronconi BM (1993) Myasthenia gravis: recognition of a human autoantigen at the molecular level. *Immunol Today* **14**: 363–368.

■ This review article discusses the immunopathology of myasthenia gravis. It describes recent research involved in characterising the response to the acetylcholine receptor and the repertoire of T cell receptor and IgH genes used.

Richman DP, Agius MA (1994) Acquired myasthenia gravis. *Immunopathol Neurol Clin* **12**(2): 273–284.

■ This article looks at the mechanism of tolerance breakdown in myasthenia gravis and discusses the potential for antigenic mimicry as a stimulus for this disease.

Rose NR, Bona C (1993) Defining criteria for autoimmune diseases (Witebsky's postulates revisited). *Immunol Today* **14**: 426–430.

■ There is some confusion over defining a disease as autoimmune. In the 1950s, criteria were established, based on Koch's postulates, which could be used for defining autoimmune diseases. Since this time, our knowledge of the cellular and molecular mechanisms involved in the immune response has expanded tremendously. This review looks at the established criteria in the light of our new knowledge and assesses the validity of the original Witebsky's postulates in defining autoimmune diseases today. It gives a rational and reasoned approach to the defining of a disease as autoimmune and clearly explains the rationale behind it. It is important to understand how such diseases are classified and this article explains it very well.

Schattner A (1994) Lymphokines in autoimmunity — a critical review. *Clin Immunol Immunopathol* **70**: 177–189.

■ Studies in recent years have implicated lymphokines in the development and exacerbation of autoimmune disease. Those shown to be particularly important include the interferons, tumour necrosis factor and interleukins-1 and -2. Indeed, raised levels of lymphokines have been demonstrated in the circulation or in relevant tissues in many patients with autoimmune disease. These raised levels often correlate with disease activity. This article discusses current evidence for a seminal role for lymphokines in autoimmune disease pathology.

Young DB (1990) The immune response to mycobacterial heat shock proteins. *Autoimmunity* **7**: 237–244.

■ The highly conserved nature of the heat shock proteins across species and their local accumulation in response to stress has led to extensive research into their involvement in autoimmunity due to molecular mimicry. This article considers the impact of this work.

Zouali M, Kalsi J, Isenberg D (1993) Autoimmune diseases — at the molecular level. *Immunol Today* **14**: 473–476.

■ This article considers the repertoire of T cell receptor genes used in autoimmune diseases, the selection and triggering of autoantibody-producing B cells and the targets for autoimmune attack. It is a general review which illustrates its arguments with a number of different autoimmune diseases.

CHAPTER 10

King CL, Nutman TB (1993) Cytokines and immediate hypersensitivity in protective immunity to helminth infections. *Infect Agents Dis* **2**: 103–108.

■ This review looks at the cytokines involved in the response to tissue-invasive helminth infection. Such infections are typically characterised by a type I hypersensitivity reaction showing IgE elevation and circulating eosinophilia.

Kovesi G (1994) Mucosal immunity. *Acta Microbiol Immunol Hung* **41**(3): 221–239.

McGhee JR, Kiyono H (1993) New perspectives in vaccine development: mucosal immunity to infections. *Infect Agents Dis* **2**: 55–73.

■ This review focuses on the unique features of the mucosal immune system and discusses how the common mucosal immune system may contain distinct compartments. It also describes the differences in antigen uptake, processing and presentation in mucosal inductive and effector sites. The review also discusses the features of the mucosal immune system which need to be considered when developing vaccines. It is a lengthy but readable review which gives a good introduction to the problems involved in developing vaccines.

Reynolds HY (1994) Respiratory host defenses — surface immunity. *Immunobiology* **191**: 402–412.

■ This is a review of the mucosal immune mechanisms which occur in the respiratory tract. It is relatively easy reading which allows you to understand the differences between the respiratory mucosal immune responses and those of digestive mucosae.

CHAPTER 11

Berke G (1994) The binding and lysis of target cells by cytotoxic lymphocytes: molecular and cellular aspects. *Annu Rev Immunol* **12**: 735–773.

■ This review covers the molecular and cellular mechanisms involved in cytotoxic T cell activity. It is a detailed review which is relatively easy to read and covers most aspects of this important method of immunity to infection.

Herman A, Kappler JW, Marrack P, Pullen AM (1991) Superantigens: mechanism of T-cell stimulation and role in immune responses. *Annu Rev Immunol* **9**: 745–772.

Kaufmann SHE (1989) Immunity to bacteria and fungi. *Curr Opin Immunol* **1**: 431–440.

■ This review of the literature current in 1989 gives a good overview of the understanding of how the host copes with infection caused by bacteria and fungi. It is easy to read and to follow.

Kaufmann SHE (1993) Immunity to intracellular bacteria. *Annu Rev Immunol* **11**: 129–163.

■ This review describes the immunological responses required for controlling intracellular bacterial infections. It discusses the role of Th subsets and cytokines and describes the role of $\gamma\delta$ T cells.

Lehrer RI, Lichtenstein AK, Ganz T (1993) Defensins: antimicrobial and cytotoxic peptides of mammalian cells. *Annu Rev Immunol* **11**: 105–128.

Sher A, Coffman RL (1992) Regulation of immunity to parasites by T cells and T cell-derived cytokines. *Annu Rev Immunol* **10**: 385–409.
∎ This review describes the roles of CD4+ and CD8+ cells in immunity to parasites. It also describes the associated pathology in diseases such as malaria, toxoplasmosis and schistosomiasis. It is well written and easy to follow.

Steller H (1995) Mechanisms and genes of cellular suicide. *Science* **267**: 1445–1449.

CHAPTER 12

Falkow S, Isberg RR, Portnoy DA (1992) The interaction of bacteria with mammalian cells. *Annu Rev Cell Biol* **8**: 333–363.

Glauser MP, Zanetti G, Baumgartner J-D, Cohen J (1991) Septic shock: pathogenesis. *Lancet* **338**: 732–739.
∎ This review describes the multifaceted effects of endotoxin which lead to the condition known as septic shock. It deals with a complex subject in a very understandable way. It is worth a read.

Joiner KA (1988) Complement evasion by bacteria and parasites. *Annu Rev Microbiol* **42**: 201–230.
∎ This review gives an overview of the complement system before describing ways in which micro-organisms can evade destruction, either directly or indirectly, by complement. It gives a description of the biochemistry of C3, explaining how it participates in both the classical and alternative pathways.

Marrack P, Kappler J (1994) Subversion of the immune system by pathogens. *Cell* **76**: 323–332.
∎ This is a relatively brief review which describes the ways in which micro-organisms avoid being destroyed by the immune system or how they use the immune response to their own advantage. It is relatively easy to read and quite straightforward.

Rook GAW (1988) Role of activated macrophages in the immunopathology of tuberculosis. *Br Med Bull* **44**: 611–623.
∎ This review describes how interferon-gamma, which activates macrophages infected by *Mycobacterium tuberculosis*, is involved in the pathology associated with the infection.

Thompson CB (1995) Apoptosis in the pathogenesis and treatment of disease. *Science* **267**: 1456–1462.
∎ Apoptosis is induced in cells by cytotoxic effector cells in virus infections but it is also involved in cell death in a number of other diseases. This review describes the diseases in which cell death is either increased or decreased.

CHAPTER 13

Hellstrom I, Helstrom KE (1993) Tumor immunology: an overview. *Ann NY Acad Sci* **690**: 24–33.

This brief review of tumour immunology covers most aspects of the subject in a readable form.

Hellstrom KE, Hellstrom I, Linsley P, Chen L (1993) On the role of costimulation in tumor immunity. *Ann NY Acad Sci* **690**: 225–230.

This is an interesting brief review by the same authors as the reference above.

Hu SL, Hellstrom I, Hellstrom KE (1992) Recent advances in antitumor vaccines. *Biotechnology* **20**: 327–343.

This article considers the role of anti-idiotypic antibodies in the destruction of human tumours. The contrasting evidence in animal studies of the role of anti-idiotypic antibodies in the inhibition of tumour growth has led to many questions which this paper tries, in some part, to answer. It is an interesting article concerning the treatment of this problematic group of diseases.

Lynch SA, Houghton AN (1993) Cancer immunology. *Curr Opin Oncol* **5**: 145–150.

In this review, the authors consider the current progress in cancer immunology. They look at the molecular identification of tumour antigens, cytokine gene transfer into cancer cells and the adoptive transfer of immune effector cells.

Miller AR, McBride WH, Hunt K, Economou JS (1994) Cytokine-mediated gene therapy for cancer. *Ann Surg Oncol* **1**: 436–450.

This article describes the potential for treatment of cancer using tumour-directed cytokine gene transfer. It describes the work which has been done with a variety of cytokine genes and the ways in which they have influenced the outcome of experimental and natural cancers.

CHAPTER 14

Clark DA (1991) Controversies in reproductive immunology. *Crit Rev Immunol* **11**: 215–247.

This lengthy review carefully and thoroughly examines the way in which pregnancy is maintained and those factors which may be involved in spontaneous abortion. It is well written and worth a read.

Clark DA, Slapsys R, Chaput A, Walker C, Brierley J, Saya S, Rosenthal KL (1986) Immunoregulatory molecules of trophoblast and decidual suppressor cell origin at the maternofetal interface. *Am J Reprod Immunol Microbiol* **10**: 100–104.

This is a relatively old article but one which explains the organisation of the decidua at both a tissue and a cellular level.

Lala PK, Kearns M (1985) Immunobiology of the decidual tissue. *Contrib Gynecol Obstet* **14**: 1–15.

■ This is a rather old but informative review of the cells associated with decidual tissue.

Lyons RM, Moses HL (1990) Transforming growth factors and the regulation of cell proliferation. *Eur J Biochem* **187**: 467.

Miyazono K, Heldin C-H (1993) The mechanism of action of transforming growth factor-*β*. *Gastroenterol Jap* **28**: S81–S85.
■ This is a concise review which describes the structure and synthesis of transforming growth factor-beta and of the receptors and regulatory proteins which control its activity.

Rifkin DB, Kohima S, Abe M, Harpel JG (1993) TGF-*β*: structure, function and formation. *Thromb Haemost* **70**: 177–179.
■ This is a brief article which describes the distinctive synthesis and secretion of this lymphokine.

Vassalli P (1992) The pathophysiology of tumor necrosis factors. *Annu Rev Immunol* **10**: 411–452.

CHAPTER 15

Charlton B, Auchincloss H, Fathman CG (1994) Mechanisms of transplantation tolerance. *Annu Rev Immunol* **12**: 707–734.
■ This review describes the tolerance mechanisms involved in acceptance of transplanted tissue. It is relevant also to the chapter on tolerance and describes fundamental mechanisms of tolerance induction. It also introduces you to the concept of chimeras. It should help you to realise how many of the mechanisms we have discussed in this book may be relevant to a number of different clinical situations and to how we treat, cure or prevent them.

Gaston RS (1994) Cytokines and transplantation: a clinical perspective. *Transplant Sci* **4**: S9–S19.
■ This review describes the role of cytokines in allograft rejection. It also looks at the therapeutic use of cytokines in transplantation.

Lafferty KJ (1994) A contemporary view of transplantation tolerance: an immunologist's perspective. *Clin Transplant* **8**: 181–187.

Storek J, Saxon A (1992) Reconstitution of B cell immunity following bone marrow transplantation. *Bone Marrow Transplant* **9**: 395–408.
■ This review looks at the occurrence of post-transplantation humoral immunodeficiency and discusses the underlying immunological mechanisms which may be involved in this condition.

CHAPTER 16

Blaese RM, Culver KW (1992) Gene therapy for primary immunodeficiency disease. *Immunodefic Rev* **3**: 329–349.
■ This review looks at the potential use of gene therapy for treatment of primary immunodeficiency diseases. The authors describe the development and preliminary

results of a gene therapy for ADA-SCID. They also discuss the potential for developing somatic cell gene therapy for other primary immunodeficiency diseases.

Cease KB, Berzofsky JA (1994) Toward a vaccine for AIDS: the emergence of immunobiology-based vaccine development. *Annu Rev Immunol* **12**: 923–989.

■ This review describes the complexities involved in developing a vaccine against AIDS. Many of the parameters considered are common to vaccine development in general. This is an interesting article which you should not find difficult to read. Try to decide how the observations made in this article could be applied to the development of vaccines for other infections. At this stage you should be able to read and appreciate the article by Arnon and van Regenmortel listed in the Further Reading for Chapter 2.

Conley ME (1992) Molecular approaches to analysis of X-linked immunodeficiencies. *Annu Rev Immunol* **10**: 215–238.

Islam KB, Baskin B, Nilsson L, Hammarstrom L, Sideras P, Smith CI (1994) Molecular analysis of IgA deficiency. Evidence for impaired switching to IgA. *J Immunol* **152**: 1442–1452.

■ This article looks at the molecular evidence for abnormal immunoglobulin gene switching in patients with IgA deficiency.

Kinnon C, Hinshelwood S, Levinsky RJ, Lovering RC (1993) X-linked agammaglobulinemia — gene cloning and future prospects. *Immunol Today* **14**: 554–558.

Klein C, Lisowska-Grospierre B, LeDeist F, Fischer A, Griscelli C (1993) Major histocompatibility complex class II deficiency: clinical manifestations, immunologic features, and outcome. *J Pediatr* **123**: 921–928.

Leonard WJ, Noguchi M, Russel SM, McBride OW (1994) The molecular basis of X-linked severe combined immunodeficiency: the role of the interleukin-2 receptor γ chain as a common j chain, jc. *Immunol Rev* **138**: 61–86.

Levy JA (1993) Pathogenesis of human immunodeficiency virus infection. *Microbiol Rev* **57**: 183–289.

■ This is an excellent review although, as with all HIV work, it is already out of date. However, it is still worth a read, due to its easy style. It will give you a good understanding of the field, from which point you should go on to read some of the seminal references covering the early observations and the recent advances.

Noguchi M, Yi H, Rosenblatt HM, Filipovich AH, Adelstein S, Modi WS, McBride OW, Leonard WJ (1993) Interleukin-2 receptor γ chain mutation results in X-linked severe combined immunodeficiency in humans. *Cell* **73**: 147–157.

Rawlings DJ, Witte ON (1994) Bruton's tyrosine kinase is a key regulator in B cell development. *Immunol Rev* **138**: 105–119.

Schaffer FM, Monteiro RC, Volanakis JE, Cooper MD (1991) IgA deficiency. *Immunodefic Rev* **3**: 15–44.

■ IgA is the most common primary immunodeficiency disease and this review describes the heterogeneous nature of this disease.

Index

Note: page numbers in *italics* refer to figures and tables

Index compiled by Jill Halliday

How to Use the Self-assessment Program

Having loaded the program according to the instructions on the disk, you should have an icon under program manager. Double click on this and the opening page will be displayed. When you have read this, you should click on OK. The test page is now displayed. In order to set up a test, click on the MCQ test button. This will display a list of chapters. Move the highlight bar over the chapter on which you wish to test yourself using the up and down arrow keys and press return (or double click on the chapter with the mouse). The test starts immediately. You answer a question either by clicking the button with the appropriate letter at the bottom of the screen or by pressing the appropriate letter key on your keyboard. If you get the correct answer, a box is displayed with the word 'correct'. Click 'OK' to continue to the next question. If you select the wrong answer, the box displayed gives an explanation of why your answer was wrong. Again, click 'OK' when you have read this. You may stop the test at any time by clicking on the 'stop now' key at the bottom of the screen. This displays your 'score card', and, by clicking on the 'print' button, you can keep a record of how well you have done. Clicking on the 'OK' button returns you to the test page.

If you click on the 'Random' button, you will notice that (off) changes to (on). This allows you to select from more than one chapter and to produce a randomised and/or timed test. Having turned on the 'random' option, clicking 'MCQ test' will display the list of chapters again. Clicking on the chapters allows you to select which chapters you wish to use (clicking them a second time deselects them). When you have made your selection, click 'OK'. A box appears which tells you how many questions are available and asks how many you wish to attempt. Type a number at the prompt and press return. The test should commence. Randomisation means that not only are the questions picked at random, but also that the answers are shuffled so that although the correct answer may be 'A' the first time you see the question, it may be 'E' the next time you see it. Again, you may stop the test at any time and the score card is displayed.

If you wish to give yourself a timed test, click the 'timed test' box on the test page and enter the length of time of the test in the 'Minutes' box. This is done by simply clicking in the box and typing the numbers. In such a test, the correct and explanation boxes are not displayed after each question and the test automatically stops when you have had the length of time selected. The 'results page' is automatically displayed and again may be printed for your records.

Finally, the configure system button allows you to alter the look of your program (by changing the font size and background colours) and its operation (by preventing interruption of a test or not showing explanations).

Try it and have some fun!

INSTALLATION INSTRUCTIONS

The disk that accompanies this book contains two files:

SETUP.EXE

and

README.TXT.

The program is installed as follows:

1. Start Microsoft Windows.
2. Insert the disk into the appropriate drive on your PC.
3. Within the *Windows Program Manager*, select *Run* . . . from the *File* Menu.
4. Enter the command *< drive >:SETUP* where *< drive >* is the letter used to identify the drive that the disk has been placed in.
5. The installation routine will install the program and will create the appropriate icons with *Program Manager*.
6. Once installation has been completed the program will automatically run.

You may experience problems printing your test results on a network running a TCP/IP network protocol.